Introduction

Acne (Figure 1) is one of the commonest skin diseases that community physicians and dermatologists have to treat. Confirming the diagnosis is rarely a problem and, given the wide spectrum of treatment options, there really is no reason why most patients with acne cannot be helped enormously. However, the vast number of therapeutic options now available can pose difficulties for the prescribing clinician in deciding which is the preferred treatment. The purpose of this guide is to highlight several features of the disease, including etiology and clinical presentation, while also reviewing the treatments available along with their respective modes of action and potential adverse effects.

Successful management of acne requires careful selection of antiacne agents according to clinical presentation and individual patient needs. A thorough patient evaluation should take into account acne severity and

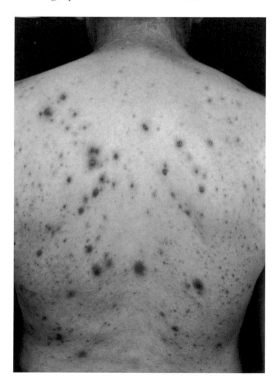

Figure 1 A typical example of common acne.

predominant lesion type as well as age, skin type, lifestyle, motivation and the presence of coexisting conditions. Incorporation of all these factors, along with appropriate education when choosing a specific treatment program, can enhance patient compliance and satisfaction, which is essential for the success of acne treatment. The recent introduction of several new antiacne agents affords greater flexibility in treatment. The availability of new treatment options to complement the existing armamentarium should help to achieve the successful therapy of greater numbers of acne patients, ensure improved tolerability and fulfill patient expectations.

1 Epidemiology

Acne can affect persons of all ages, including neonates, infants, prepubescent children, adolescents and mature adults. However, acne is most prevalent and most severe during adolescence.

Neonatal acne (Figure 1.1) is characterized by the development of comedones, and inflammatory papules and pustules which generally affect the cheeks. It is thought to result from the production of androgens by the fetal adrenal glands and testes. Neonatal acne usually resolves within the first 3 months of life, but can persist for up to a year.

In females, acne becomes active again at the time of adrenarche, generally around 8 to 10 years of age. The onset of acne in this period has been associated with elevated levels of dehydroepiandrosterone sulfate (DHEAS), a weak adrenal androgen. Most prepubertal acne is characterized by the presence of comedones and few inflammatory lesions.

Acne vulgaris typically begins around puberty and early adolescence; thus it tends to present earlier in females than males, reaching peak severity in females at about the age of 17, and at 19 or 20 years in

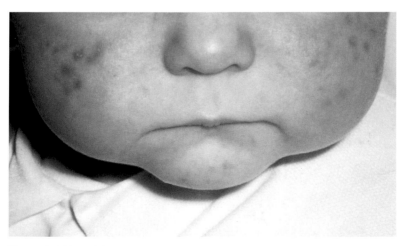

Figure 1.1 Neonatal acne.

males. The face is usually the first site to be affected, but later the trunk will be significantly involved in about 30% of patients. In some patients the acne may be localized to one site such as the chin or forehead or upper part of the back or chest; in others, all sites are equally affected.

Most adolescents will have a little acne – often referred to as physiological acne. Estimates of the prevalence of acne in the adolescent age group approach 100%. The point at which mild physiological acne becomes clinical acne is not very well defined, as there is frequently a continuous spectrum of severity. Examples of facial acne graded according to the Leeds Grading System can be found on pages 76–9.

Duration of acne and its resolution

Physiological acne usually lasts only a few years. Clinical acne may last well into the 20s, usually up to about 25 years of age, but acne will persist for longer in some 7% of individuals; if acne is evident up to 30 years of age it is likely to persist until age 45. Acne can even affect postmenopausal women, where it is thought to result from unopposed androgen secretion by the ovaries. Whether the increased incidence of mature or persistent acne is a new phenomenon or this clinical presentation has simply been more recently recognized is uncertain. The reason for the eventual decline in the prevalence of acne with age is also unknown, but is thought possibly to relate to the decline in serum DHEAS levels associated with the aging process.

Key points – epidemiology

- Acne vulgaris typically occurs around adolescence.
- Acne vulgaris can present in the neonate, and it can persist beyond adolescence in susceptible individuals.
- Physiological acne, i.e. very mild acne, is considered a normal variant of maturation.
- Clinical acne persists and progresses beyond the period of adolescence.
- Acne persisting beyond 25 years of age is likely to persist for a further 10–20 years.

Key references

Cunliffe WJ, Gollnick HPM. *Acne – Diagnosis and Management*. London: Martin Dunitz, 2001.

Goulden V, Clark SM, Cunliffe WJ. Post-adolescent acne: a review of clinical features. *Br J Dermatol* 1997;136:66–70.

Herane MI, Ando I. Acne in infancy and acne genetics. *Dermatology* 2003;206:24–8.

Katsambas AD, Katoulis AC, Stravopoulos P. Acne neonatorum: a study of 22 cases. *Int J Dermatol* 1999;38:128–30.

Lucky AW, Biro FM, Huster GA et al. Acne vulgaris in premenarchal girls. *Arch Dermatol* 1994;130:308–14.

The pathophysiology of acne centers on the interplay of increased
sebum production, follicular hyperkeratinization, the action of
Propionibacterium acnes (*P. acnes*) within the follicle, and the
production of inflammation (Figure 2.1). It is a hormonally mediated
disease with androgens playing a role both in controlling sebum
production by the sebaceous gland and in influencing follicular
hyperkeratinization. Acne patients are not hormonal misfits – most
patients with acne are hormonally well. Only infrequently do women
with acne suffer from irregular menses or hirsutism. The increased
sebum production, which correlates well with acne severity, presents
as seborrhea.

Comedones are due to follicular hyperkeratinization and possibly
also to an increase in cell division and cohesiveness of the cells lining
the follicular lumen. This process has been referred to as 'follicular
plugging', although complete occlusion of the follicular lumen does not
occur – sebum still flows from follicles affected with acne. The cause
of follicular hyperkeratinization is not known but may relate to a
local deficiency of linoleic acid, production of cytokines such as
interleukin-1 within the follicle, or possibly the effects of androgens
on keratinization. Once sebum production begins at adrenarche,
sebaceous follicles become colonized with *P. acnes*. This bacterium
utilizes sebaceous lipids as a nutrient source and hydrolyzes the
triglycerides found in sebum into free fatty acids and glycerol. The free
fatty acids are an irritant to the follicular wall and can lead to rupture
of the follicle, with subsequent release of keratin-rich corneocytes and
sebum into the dermis. This process intensifies the inflammation
associated with acne. Sebum production and sebaceous gland growth
are under the control of androgens. Dihydrotestosterone (DHT) is
thought to be the main target androgen responsible for sebum
production, although a possible direct role of testosterone in this
process has not been excluded.

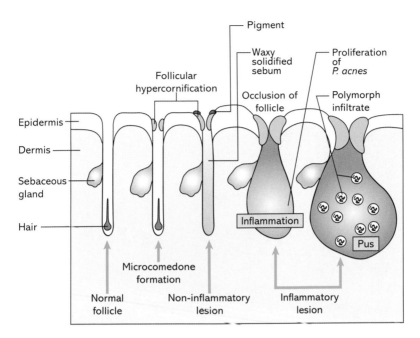

Figure 2.1 Evolution of acne within a follicle.

Microcomedones. The precursor lesion of acne is the microcomedone. This forms as a result of hyperkeratinization of the cells lining the orifice of sebaceous follicles of the face, scalp, chest or back. (A microcomedone is not clinically visible but can be identified by the technique of surface follicular biopsy using cyanoacrylate glue applied to a glass microscope slide.) As hyperkeratinization progresses, a microcomedone develops into either an open or closed comedone: a blackhead or whitehead, respectively. It takes approximately 8 weeks for a microcomedone to develop into a visible acne lesion. This is one reason why the full effect of acne medications is not achieved until therapy has been administered for several weeks.

Inflammatory lesions develop from comedones following the influx of inflammatory cells and/or rupture of the follicular wall. Recent studies demonstrate the involvement of inflammatory responses even in the very earliest phases of development of acne lesions and show that sebocytes, acting as immune cells, may play a role in the development of microcomedones. Interestingly, cutaneous neurogenic factors too, such as Substance P, may contribute to the onset and/or exacerbation of acne inflammation. The lesions may evolve into tender inflammatory nodules or 'cysts' as the extent of the inflammation increases. Inflammatory acne may produce acne scarring. Scarring can be due to loss of tissue, as in atrophic scars (Figure 2.2) or ice-pick scars (Figure 2.3), or due to an increase in tissue as in hypertrophic or fibrotic scars (Figure 2.4).

Modifying factors

Certain myths still remain about factors that might influence the disease (Table 2.1). The appropriate facts need to be shared with the patient. For example, acne is not influenced by food. It is frequently worse before the menstrual period. Stress may worsen acne; in turn, acne certainly and frequently causes more stress. Natural sunshine often helps acne, but if the sunshine is associated with sweating, particularly in an area of high humidity, then the acne frequently flares. This flare is likely to be the result of partial blocking of the sebaceous gland pores by sweat.

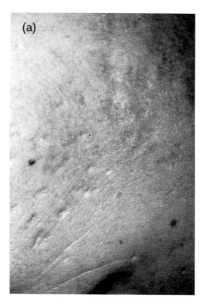
(a)

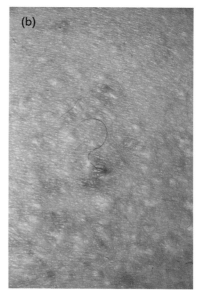
(b)

Figure 2.2 (a) Macular atrophic scars: soft distensible scars on face.
(b) Perifollicular elastolysis on trunk.

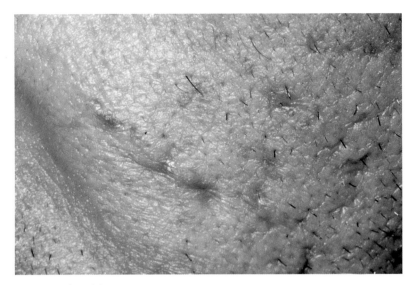

Figure 2.3 Ice-pick scars.

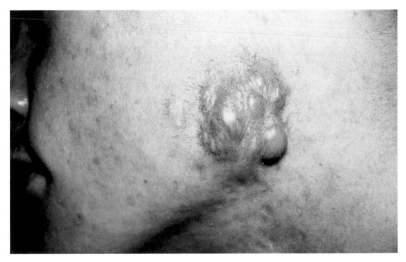

Figure 2.4 Hypertrophic scarring on angle of jaw.

Acne often occurs at an age when an individual is experiencing many significant psychological and social changes. Thus, not infrequently, acne will lead to loss of self-esteem, anxiety, problems with mixing with peers and, at times, significant depression. Not uncommonly, acne produces a loss of motivation in carrying out day-to-day activities; such activities may include shopping, going away for a weekend or holidays, going out to socialize at the pub, night club, discos or even simply for a meal. Patients with acne also have greater employment difficulties than the general population; in one survey, 22% of respondents believed that they had been turned down for a job because of their skin.

In some studies of patients with severe acne, the levels of social, psychological and emotional problems were as great as those reported by patients with conditions such as chronic disabling asthma, epilepsy, diabetes, back pain or arthritis. Depression and suicidal ideation has been studied in dermatology patients with a variety of skin conditions, including acne. The incidence of suicidal ideation found in 72 patients with mild-to-moderate acne was 5.6%. This was higher than the 2.4–3.3% prevalence reported among general medical patients.

For many patients, the psychological and social effects of acne motivate them to seek professional consultation and treatment. Because acne does not affect patients in terms of their general medical health, if the psychosocial effect of the condition is not fully appreciated by a patient's parent or physician, acne could be easily dismissed as merely a cosmetic problem. It is important for the physician to realize that there is tremendous variation among individuals in the degree of psychological distress produced by acne. In some cases, physicians may be dismissive about a mild case of acne; however, the patient may exhibit significant psychopathology. In fact, many studies have shown that a patient's dissatisfaction with their facial appearance significantly correlates with *their* rating of their acne severity and not with the rating determined by the physician. Several studies performed in acne patients before and after treatment have documented improvements in a wide variety of psychological functions as a result of successful treatment. In many patients, the psychosocial disability caused by acne can be reversed with effective treatment.

There are a number of disease-specific questionnaires that can be used to assess the psychological impact of acne, e.g. Assessments of Psychosocial Effects of Acne (APSEA; see Figure 8.1 on page 68), the Cardiff Acne Disability Index (CADI) or the Dermatology Quality of Life Index (DQLI). It is important to consider the psychosocial morbidity of the disease when considering treatment.

Acne scarring (see pages 12–13) can also cause significant disfigurement and correlates with psychological problems. It is also very difficult to treat (see pages 65–6). Its identification is an important part of the initial assessment. Apparent scarring should be taken into consideration when deciding on the treatment regimen.

Dysmorphophobia is a recognized psychological condition seen in patients with very minimal facial acne. The patient's perception of their clinical acne problem is significantly out of proportion to the real skin disease evident. There is frequently an association with clinical depression and/or an obsessional neurosis. Any acne should be treated, but ideally management should be conducted in collaboration with a psychiatrist, psychologist or counselor where practical.

Key points – psychosocial aspects

- Acne and scarring can cause significant psychosocial disability.
- Psychological changes should be noted and taken into account when treating acne.
- Validated and recognized questionnaires are available to assess the psychological disability produced by acne.
- Dysmorphophobia is frequently associated with depression and/or obsessional neurosis. Psychiatric input is invaluable.
- Acne excoriée may be alleviated by habit reversal therapy.

Acne excoriée (see Figure 4.12 on page 29) frequently occurs in adolescent girls and young women. A proportion of patients have primary underlying inflammatory acne and/or an atopic background. Patients pick and scratch, leading to exacerbation of lesions. Treatment can be difficult. The importance of not picking must be emphasized. Habit reversal techniques have been successfully used. Oral pimozide has been used with some success. Acne should be treated, if present, with a conventional approach.

Key references

Cotterill JA. Dermatologic nondisease. *Dermatol Clin* 1996;14:409–45.

Cunliffe WJ. Unemployment and acne. *Br J Dermatol* 1986;1115:386.

Finlay AY, Khan CK. Dermatology Life Quality Index (DLQI) – a simple practical measure for routine clinical use. *Clin Exp Dermatol* 1992;17:1–3.

Gupta MA, Gupta AK. Depression and suicide ideation in dermatology patients with acne, alopecia areata, atopic dermatitis and psoriasis. *Br J Dermatol* 1998;139:846–50.

Kellet S, Gawkrodger DJ. The psychological and emotional impact of chronic acne and the effect of treatment with isotretinoin. *Br J Dermatol* 1998;139(suppl):51–6.

Kent A, Drummond LM. Acne excoriée – a case report using habit reversal. *Clin Exp Dermatol* 1989;14:163–4.

Layton AM, Seukaran DC, Cunliffe WJ. Scarred for life. *Dermatology* 1997;195:15–21.

Layton AM. Acne scarring – reviewing the need for early treatment of acne. *J Dermatol Treat* 2000;11:3–6.

Motley RJ, Finlay AJ. Practical use of a disability index in the routine management of acne. *Clin Exp Dermatol* 1992;17(1):1–3.

Newton J. The effectiveness of acne treatment: an assessment by patients of outcome of treatment. *Br J Dermatol* 1997;137(4):563–7.

Niemeier V, Kupfer J, Demmelbauer-Ebner M et al. Coping with acne vulgaris. *Dermatology* 1998;196:108–15.

Seukaran DC, Cunliffe WJ, Islam J. The psychological impact of acne scarring. *Br J Dermatol* 1999;144(suppl):154–5.

Sneddon J, Sneddon I. Acne excoriée: a protective device. *Clin Exp Dermatol* 1983;8:65–8.

Clinical features of the various forms of acne

Lesion types

Acne vulgaris is the most common type of acne. Other types are described later in this chapter. The individual lesions of acne vulgaris are divisible into three types:

- non-inflamed lesions
- inflamed lesions
- scars.

Non-inflamed lesions are called comedones. Comedones may be microscopic (microcomedones) (Figure 4.1) or evident to the eye as blackheads or whiteheads (Figure 4.2). Microcomedones, the precursor lesions of acne, may develop into whiteheads or blackheads.

- Whiteheads (closed comedones) are small spots (about 1 mm in size) and are usually white or cream in color. Macrocomedones are large closed comedones, usually > 2 mm in diameter, and are usually white in color and palpable (Figure 4.3).

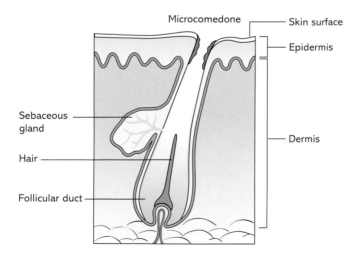

Figure 4.1 A microcomedone, the precursor lesion of acne.

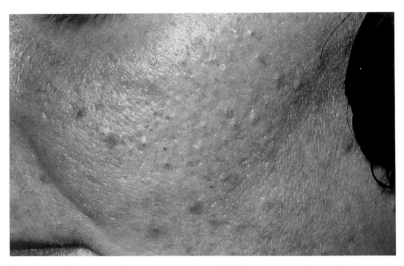

Figure 4.2 Mixed non-inflammatory lesions: blackheads and whiteheads.

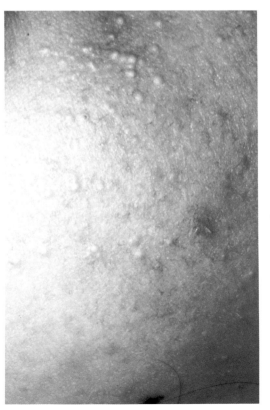

Figure 4.3
Macrocomedones: closed comedones of diameter > 2 mm.

- Blackheads (open comedones) are of similar size and really need no description. The reason for the black appearance is the presence of the skin pigment melanin which has undergone oxidation.

Open and closed comedones need to be distinguished because, in closed comedones, the contents of the pore cannot escape as easily (their external orifice is very small) as from an open comedone. Thus, closed comedones, like microcomedones and macrocomedones, are more likely to become inflamed. Most patients have a mixture of non-inflamed and inflamed lesions.

Inflamed lesions may be superficial (papules, pustules) or deep pustules or nodules (Figure 4.4). Papules are small, raised, red spots (< 0.5 cm); superficial pustules are of a similar size and predominantly yellow (Figure 4.5). Nodules are larger lesions (> 0.6 cm) and are deeper; they persist much longer (2–3 weeks) than papules and

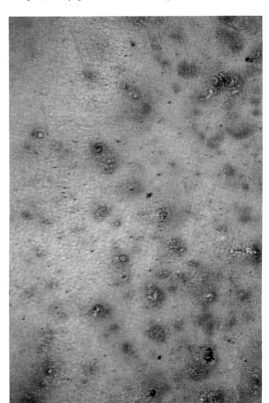

Figure 4.4 Mixed inflammatory and non-inflammatory acne lesions.

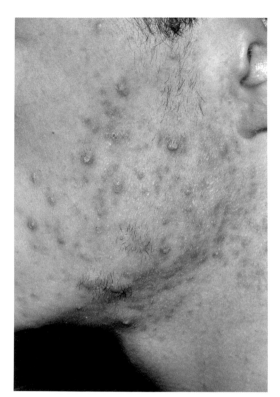

Figure 4.5 Pustular acne on the cheek.

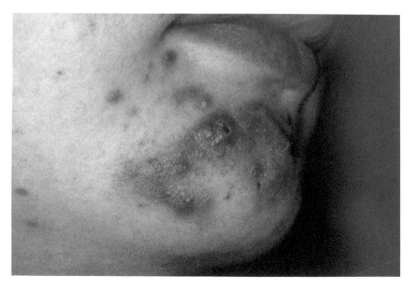

Figure 4.6 Acne nodule: an inflammatory lesion of diameter > 6 mm.

pustules, which last 7–10 days. Nodules (Figure 4.6) are often firm initially and may be tender, but as the inflammation develops they frequently soften.

Scars. Nodules are associated with scarring in many cases, but even papular or pustular acne lesions can lead to scars. Increased accumulation of dermal collagen may produce hypertrophic or keloid scars, especially on the angle of the jaw and the upper back and the chest (see Figure 2.4 on page 13). Such scars are firm; hypertrophic scars do not extend beyond the initial area of inflammation, while keloid scars do. Loss of dermal tissue results in large atrophic scars – especially seen on the upper trunk – or smaller but deeper ice-pick scars, especially seen on the cheek (see Figure 2.3 on page 13).

Hyperpigmentation. In some patients, particularly those with type III/IV skin, hyperpigmented macules (Figure 4.7) may persist following resolution of inflammatory acne lesions. At times, patients consider these resolving lesions to be active acne lesions and may have the erroneous impression that their acne is not improving. It is important to point out to the patient that these dark areas are healing lesions

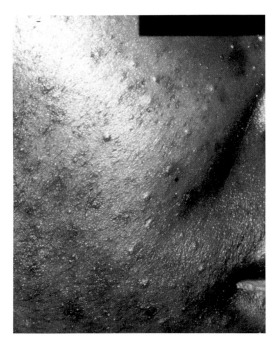

Figure 4.7
Postinflammatory
hyperpigmented macules.

and not active acne. Postinflammatory hyperpigmentation generally resolves slowly with time but may take up to a year or longer in many cases. The best solution to the problem of acne scarring and postinflammatory hyperpigmentation is to institute appropriate therapy early in the course of acne to avoid these complications.

Other forms of acne

Acne conglobata (Figure 4.8) is a very severe form of inflammatory acne characterized by grouped comedones, cysts, abscesses, draining sinus tracts and scars. The majority of affected patients are males who present with lesions involving the back, buttocks, chest and face. The axilla and inguinal areas can also be involved, producing what is called hidradenitis suppurativa. The grouped comedones often have multiple openings. The inflammatory lesions are large, tender, red to violaceous in color and often drain a serous or purulent material. Deep-seated sinus tracts often develop, as does keloidal scarring. Secondary infection with staphylococci or streptococci can occur, although many lesions are colonized only by *P. acnes*. Patients with this very severe form of

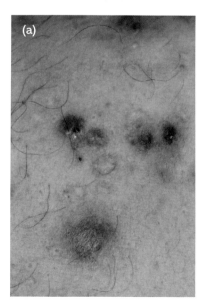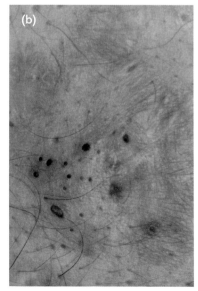

Figure 4.8 Acne conglobata: (a) deep-seated nodular acne; (b) deep-seated inflammatory lesions with grouped comedones.

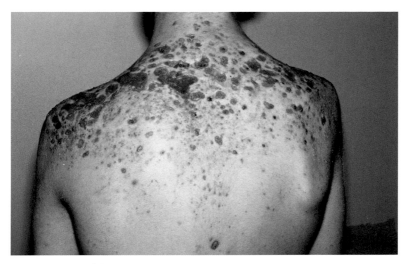

Figure 4.9 Acne fulminans.

acne require expert care with oral isotretinoin, oral and intralesional corticosteroids and surgical excision of sinus tracts. Chronicity for many years is a feature, as is poor response to therapy.

Acne fulminans (Figure 4.9) is a very severe form of inflammatory acne associated with systemic signs and symptoms including fever, arthralgias, and/or osteolytic lesions of the clavicles or ribs. It usually occurs in boys aged 13–18 years and can be very acute in its onset. Investigations frequently demonstrate leukocytosis, elevated erythrocyte sedimentation rate and/or proteinuria. Clinically, acne fulminans is characterized by multiple intensely inflamed nodules, cysts and plaques. Large nodules can ulcerate, drain and become necrotic. Hemorrhagic crusting is common. A polyarthritis of large joints such as the sacroiliac, hip, knees, shoulders, elbows and ankles may be present. The etiology of acne fulminans is unknown. Patients with this disorder should be urgently referred to a dermatologist for management with oral corticosteroids and isotretinoin (Table 4.1).

Acne with solid facial edema. In rare cases, acne can be accompanied by a firm, non-pitting edema of the midportion of the face and forehead (Figure 4.10). The etiology of this phenomenon is unknown but may relate to lymphatic obstruction secondary to the inflammatory response associated with the acne. A primary hypoplastic

TABLE 4.1

Unusual forms of acne – suggested treatment regimens

Acne fulminans (see page 25)	• Systemic prednisone (prednisolone in UK) 0.5–1 mg/kg/day for 4–6 weeks
	• Isotretinoin 0.5 mg/kg/day after 3–4 weeks, to reach a cumulative dose of 150 mg/kg
	• Continue isotretinoin for 6–8 months
Pyoderma faciale (see page 32)	• Systemic prednisone 1 mg/kg/day for 4–6 weeks
	• Daily application of type IV topical corticosteroid for 1 week (optional to reduce inflammation)
	• Oral isotretinoin 0.25–0.5 mg/kg/day introduced after 1 week, gradually increasing to 1 mg/kg/day in next 3–4 weeks
	• Continue isotretinoin therapy
Gram-negative folliculitis (see page 34)	• Oral isotretinoin 0.5–1 mg/kg/day for 4–8 months

abnormality of the lymphatics is the likely cause. This condition is unresponsive to oral antibiotics but has been treated successfully at times with oral isotretinoin and corticosteroids.

Adult female acne. Adult acne, particularly in females, is worthy of special note. Although it is generally less severe than teenage acne, acne in adult women is challenging to treat. This form of acne is often characterized by tender inflammatory papules or nodules involving the lower third of the face and neck (Figure 4.11). There may also be comedonal acne involving the forehead or lateral margins of the face.

If an adult woman has a sudden onset of severe acne or if the acne is accompanied by signs of hyperandrogenism, a medical history and physical examination directed towards eliciting symptoms or signs of hyperandrogenism should be performed and investigations to rule out an underlying endocrine abnormality carried out (Table 4.2).

Screening tests for hyperandrogenism include serum DHEAS, total

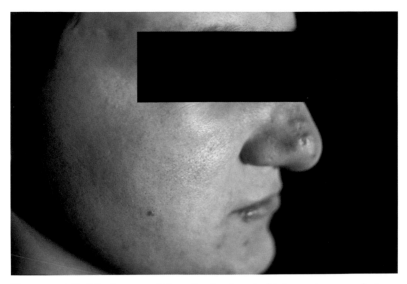

Figure 4.10 Facial edema persisting after treatment of inflammatory acne lesions.

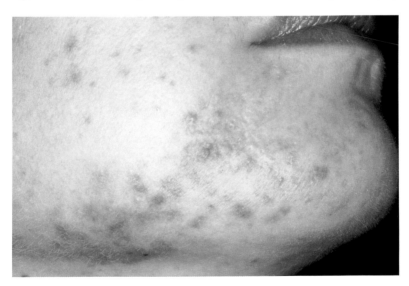

Figure 4.11 Adult, late-onset, female inflammatory acne on the chin.

testosterone, free testosterone, and luteinizing hormone / follicle-stimulating hormone (LH/FHS) ratio. These tests should be obtained in the luteal phase of the menstrual cycle (within 2 weeks prior to the onset of menses). Women should not take oral contraceptives for at

TABLE 4.2

Endocrine causes of acne

Cause	Investigations
Iatrogenic	Check family history of acne, hirsutism
Polycystic ovary syndrome	Serum testosterone, LH/FSH ratio
Congenital adrenal hyperplasia (CAH)	17(OH)-progesterone may be elevated in classic CAH, while δ-4-androstenedione is usually increased at the same time as other androgens and will not differentiate between ovarian or adrenal source. ACTH stimulation test might help identify late-onset CAH
Cushing's syndrome	Dexamethasone suppression test will help identify Cushing's syndrome or CAH
Gonadal or adrenal tumors	Serum testosterone, DHEAS
Precocious puberty	

ACTH, adrenal corticotropic hormone; DHEAS, dehydroepiandrosterone sulfate; FSH, follicle-stimulating hormone; LH, luteinizing hormone

least 1 month before the laboratory testing is performed, as these drugs can mask an underlying endocrine abnormality. Excess androgens may be produced by either the adrenal gland or the ovary. Serum DHEAS can be used to screen for an adrenal source of excess androgen production. An ovarian source of excess androgens may be suspected in cases where the serum total testosterone is elevated or the LH/FSH ratio is increased. There is significant variation in an individual's serum androgen levels. In cases where abnormal results are obtained, it is recommended that the test be repeated before proceeding with therapy or a more extensive work-up. Women with hyperandrogenism may also have insulin resistance; they are at risk for the development of diabetes and cardiovascular disease. It is therefore important for the long-term health of these patients to identify hyperandrogenism so that appropriate therapy from an endocrinologist or gynecologist can be initiated. However it needs to be stressed that in most adult females the

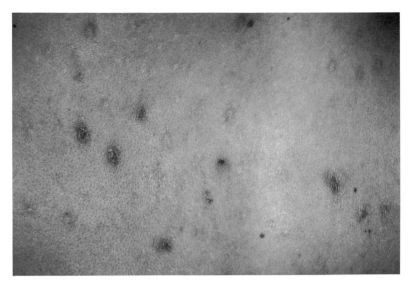

Figure 4.12 Acne excoriee: exacerbation of acne lesions by scratching.

acne represents a persistence of adolescent acne, and an endocrine work-up is rarely necessary.

Acne excoriée (Figure 4.12) is described on page 18.

Acne mechanica. Repetitive rubbing or friction over an area of skin can sometimes exacerbate acne. This is most commonly observed with sports equipment such as football helmets, shoulder pads and chin straps. It can also occur in response to habits of rubbing the face or resting the head on the hands. Acne mechanica tends to occur in cases of moderate-to-severe inflammatory acne and less often in cases of mild acne. Treatment is aimed at controlling the underlying acne and minimizing the mechanical stress on the skin.

Occupational acne. Exposure to certain industrial agents can lead to the development of acne. Coal tar derivatives and insoluble cutting oils can produce an inflammatory acne characterized by large comedones, papules, pustules, cysts and nodules. Lesions are most commonly noted in areas covered by clothing that was saturated with the offending agent.

Chloracne is caused by exposure to halogenated hydrocarbons either by ingestion, inhalation or contact with the skin. Most cases have been reported as a result of accidental industrial exposure, ingestion of contaminated food products, chemical warfare or exposure to herbicides. Implicated chemicals include polyhalogenated naphthalenes, biphenyls, dibenzofurans, dioxins and azabenzenes. Chloracne (Figure 4.13) is characterized by the development of dense collections of comedones on the face, retroauricular skin, neck, axilla and scrotum. Comedones can eventually develop into tender, inflamed cysts. Outbreaks of severe inflammatory lesions which heal with scarring can occur for years following exposure to the offending agent. Treatments include topical tretinoin and isotretinoin; physical treatment with gentle cautery under local anesthesia with EMLA cream (eutectic mixture of local anesthetics) can be particularly helpful.

Differential diagnosis of acne

The differential diagnosis of acne includes drug-induced acneiform eruptions, rosacea, pyoderma faciale, Gram-negative folliculitis, and perioral dermatitis.

Drug-induced acneiform eruptions are uncommon, but eruptions can be induced by drugs, such as anabolic and catabolic steroids, aminopterine, phenytoin, lithium, isonicotinic acid hydrazine (INH),

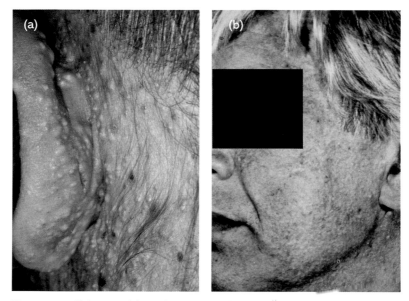

Figure 4.13 Chloracne: (a) on the retroauricular skin; (b) on the face.

TABLE 4.3

Drug-induced acne

Age of onset	Cause
Neonatal acne	Maternal ingestion of • steroids • lithium • phenytoin
Childhood acne	Direct ingestion of • steroids • dactinomycin • ciclosporin
Adolescent acne	Direct ingestion of • steroids • lithium • phenytoin • isonicotinic acid hydrazine • 8-methoxypsoralen + UVA • thiourea • thiouracil • iodides/bromides • disulfiram • quinine • azathioprine • ciclosporin A Inhaled steroid

8-methoxypsoralen + ultraviolet A light (PUVA), phenobarbitone, thiourea, thiouracil, iodides, bromides, disulfiram, quinine and azathioprine (Table 4.3). These eruptions are often sudden in onset and are characterized by inflammatory papules and pustules that are generally monomorphous in their appearance. In contrast, the lesions of acne vulgaris are a mixture of comedones, papules and pustules. Acneiform eruptions due to systemic or even inhaled steroids most commonly occur on the chest and back of hospitalized patients receiving intravenous dexamethasone, but they also occur in patients receiving high doses of oral corticosteroids and have been reported with inhaled steroids (Figure 4.14).

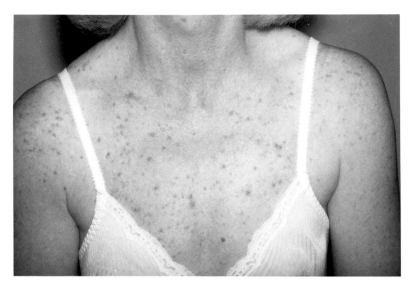

Figure 4.14 Inhaled steroid acne.

The use of topical steroids on the face can cause acneiform eruptions. Steroid-induced facial acne often develops as a secondary phenomenon during treatment of facial conditions such as eczema or seborrheic dermatitis. It presents as an increase in facial erythema and the development of inflammatory papules and pustules. Steroid acne is usually localized to discrete regions where the steroids were applied. Drug-induced acneiform eruptions resolve spontaneously following removal of the offending agent. This is not usually the case, however, with anabolic-steroid-induced acne, which is an increasing cause of such acne. Often oral isotretinoin is required to treat such patients.

Rosacea (Figure 4.15) occurs most commonly in adults with fair skin and light hair and eye color. Comedones are notably absent. It is characterized by facial flushing, erythema of the cheeks, nose, forehead and chin. Inflammatory papules and pustules can develop within the areas of erythema. In late stages of rosacea, a bulbous hypertrophy of the nose, termed rhinophyma (Figure 4.16), may occur.

Pyoderma faciale (Figure 4.17) is deemed to be an explosive form of rosacea, analogous to acne fulminans. This disorder occurs most commonly in young women with a phenotype typical

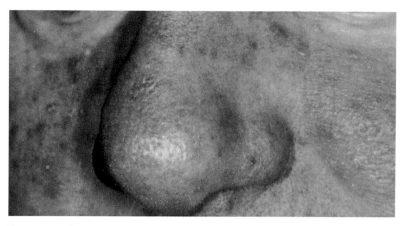

Figure 4.15 Rosacea.

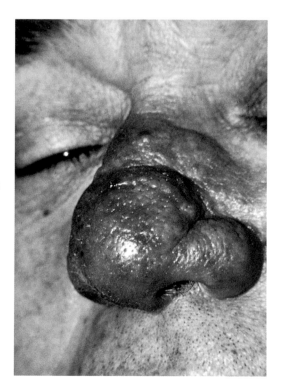

Figure 4.16 Rhinophyma
in rosacea.

of rosacea patients, often in the context of stress. Continuous
treatment with oral isotretinoin and corticosteroids is indicated
(Table 4.1).

33

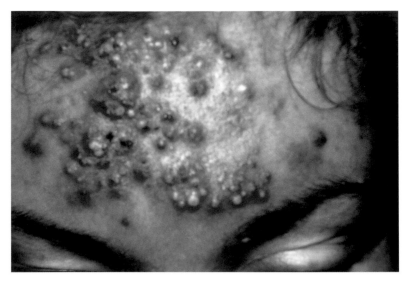

Figure 4.17 Pyoderma faciale.

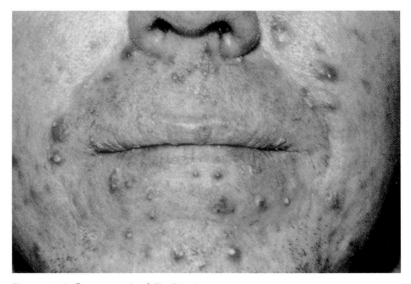

Figure 4.18 Gram-negative folliculitis.

Gram-negative folliculitis is characterized by the sudden development of superficial pustules in patients who have been treated for acne with antibiotics (Figure 4.18). It may seem to represent a flare of the underlying acne, but it is actually a folliculitis caused by Gram-

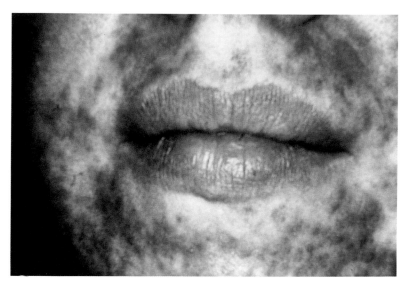

Figure 4.19 Perioral dermatitis.

negative bacteria including *Pseudomonas* and Enterobacteriaceae. Cultures of pustules should be obtained. If Gram-negative organisms are present, the patient should be referred to a dermatologist for consultation regarding treatment with isotretinoin (see Table 4.1 on page 26).

Perioral dermatitis (Figure 4.19) is characterized by erythema, scaling and small papules and pustules occurring most commonly around the mouth and on the chin. It often occurs in adult women, especially in the context of stress. Topical corticosteroids can exacerbate the condition and should be avoided. Treatment of choice is oral tetracycline.

Key points – clinical features

- Acne presents with both inflammatory and comedonal lesions in most patients.
- Acne scarring is a very common sequel to acne.
- Postinflammatory hyperpigmentation may persist for many months in type III/IV skins following the resolution of acne.
- Late-onset acne in females may relate to hyperandrogenism.
- Drugs, cosmetics, industrial agents and friction may all contribute to acne.
- Differential diagnoses of acne include rosacea, pyoderma faciale, Gram-negative folliculitis and perioral dermatitis.

Key references

Basler RS. Acne mechanica in athletes. *Cutis* 1992;50:125–8.

Bettoli V, Trimurti S, Lombardi AR, Virgili A. Acne due to amineptine abuse. *J Eur Acad Dermatol Venereol* 1998;10:281–3.

Caputo R, Monti M, Ermacora E et al. Cutaneous manifestations of tetrachlorodibenzo-p-dioxin in children and adolescents: follow-up 10 years after the Seveso, Italy, accident. *J Am Acad Dermatol* 1988;19:812–19.

Goulden V, Clark SM, Cunliffe WJ. Post adolescence acne: a review of clinical features. *Br J Dermatol* 1997;136:66–70.

Jansen T, Altmeyer P, Plewig G. Acne inversa (alias hydradenitis suppurativa). *J Eur Acad Dermatol Venereol* 2001;15:532–40.

Karvonen SL. Acne fulminans: report of clinical findings and treatment of 24 patients. *J Am Acad Dermatol* 1993;28:572–9.

Plewig G, Jansen T, Kligman A. Pyoderma faciale. A review and report of 20 additional cases: is it rosacea? *Arch Dermatol* 1992; 128:1611–17.

Poli F, Dreno B, Verschoore M. An epidemiological study of acne in female adults: results of a survey conducted in France. *J Eur Acad Dermatol Venereol* 2001;15:541–5.

Tosti A, Guerra L, Bettoli V, Bonelli U. Solid facial edema as a complication of acne vulgaris in twins. *J Am Acad Dermatol* 1987;17:843–4.

Topical therapy may be useful:
- in mild acne
- in moderate acne, in combination with oral therapy
- as maintenance therapy after stopping oral antibiotics or oral contraceptives.

Mild acne consisting of open and closed comedones and/or few inflammatory lesions is amenable to topical therapy with agents such as salicylic acid, retinoids, azelaic acid, benzoyl peroxide and topical antibiotics. Topical agents differ in their efficacy against the various etiologic factors (Table 5.1). Salicylic acid, retinoids, azelaic acid and possibly benzoyl peroxide are most effective for comedones. Benzoyl peroxide, azelaic acid, and topical antibiotics such as erythromycin, clindamycin and sodium sulfacetamide are most effective for inflammatory lesions. Retinoids and combination preparations can be used to treat non-inflammatory and inflammatory lesions.

Often patients seek medical attention for their acne after having tried a variety of over-the-counter products. Over-the-counter acne products are available as soaps, scrubs, creams, lotions and gels. Active ingredients include benzoyl peroxide, salicylic acid and α-hydroxy acids.

Benzoyl peroxide

Benzoyl peroxide releases free oxygen radicals in the sebaceous follicles, which have potent bactericidal activity against *P. acnes*. It reduces bacterial colonization of the follicle and therefore reduces the number of inflammatory lesions that develop. In addition, benzoyl peroxide decreases follicular hyperkeratosis and microcomedone formation. *P. acnes* does not develop resistance to benzoyl peroxide. For this reason, this drug is a valuable component of any acne regimen. Benzoyl peroxide is available in both over-the-counter and prescription formulations, including bar soaps, washes, gels and lotions. It is available in concentrations of 2.5%, 4%, 5% and 10%; however, there

TABLE 5.1

Topical therapies* for acne – impact on etiologic factors

	Inflammation	Comedogenesis	Reduction in *P. acnes*
Benzoyl peroxide	++	+	+++
Retinoids			
– tretinoin	+	+++	+/–
– isotretinoin	+	+++	+/–
– adapalene	+	+++	+/–
– tazarotene	+	+++	+/–
Antibiotics			
– erythromycin	++	+/–	++
– tetracycline†	++	+/–	++
– clindamycin	++	+/–	++
Combination therapies			
– zinc/erythromycin	++	+	++
– benzoyl peroxide / erythromycin	++	+	++
– isotretinoin / erythromycin	++	+	+

* The agents shown are those for which there exists adequate evidence of their action
† Not used in the USA

is no evidence that higher concentrations are more effective, and they may be more irritant. Benzoyl peroxide is generally used as a sole treatment but is available in some combination products (see page 41).

Topical retinoids

Tretinoin, or all-*trans*-retinoic acid, is a retinoid that reverses the altered keratinization in follicles affected by acne. By inhibiting the formation of the microcomedone, tretinoin prevents the development of comedones and early inflammatory lesions. Tretinoin is available as a cream, gel or solution in a variety of concentrations which differ in their potency. A rank order of potency from least to greatest would be 0.025% cream, 0.01% gel, 0.05% cream, 0.025% gel, 0.1% cream and 0.05% solution. The 0.01% gel and 0.05% cream are roughly equal in their potency, as are the 0.025% gel and 0.1% cream. Tretinoin is usually applied once daily after the face has had adequate time to dry. Tretinoin has recently become available in formulations with novel delivery systems. One such product, Retin A Micro, contains inert microspheres that have been impregnated with tretinoin. In another product, Avita, the tretinoin is incorporated within a polyoylprepolymer (PP-2). Each of these formulations releases tretinoin slowly within the follicle and onto the surface of the skin. It is thought that this slow release helps to minimize irritancy (i.e. the erythema and scaling associated with topical tretinoin). The choice of vehicle for tretinoin delivery depends upon whether the patient has dry or oily skin. Gels are usually preferred by patients with oily skin, and creams are preferred by patients with dry skin.

Adapalene is a synthetic acid derivative with retinoid-like activity but a distinctly different chemical structure. Adapalene is a potent modulator of cellular differentiation, keratinization and inflammatory processes, whose mechanism of action is believed to be similar to that of retinoids. Adapalene interacts with nuclear retinoic acid receptors (RARs) and is selective for RARβ and RARγ. Adapalene does not interact with retinoid X receptors (RXRs). It has been hypothesized that this receptor selectivity may account for differences in its side-effect profile.

Adapalene has been shown to possess anti-inflammatory activity in a number of in-vitro and in-vivo animal models. Clinical studies have demonstrated adapalene 0.1% gel to be as effective in the treatment of acne as tretinoin 0.025% cream and to be less irritant and with a faster mode of action. It is available as a 0.1% gel and 0.1% solution for the treatment of acne.

Tazarotene is a synthetic acetylenic retinoid that has been formulated into a topical gel and studied for its safety and efficacy in acne and psoriasis. Following topical application, tazarotene is converted to its active metabolite, tazarotenic acid. This compound then binds to nuclear RARs and can affect expression of genes involved in cell proliferation, cell differentiation and inflammation. At the cellular level this may result in a modification of several pathogenic factors in acne, including corneocyte accumulation and cohesion. Tazarotene is specific for RARs compared with RXRs and selectively activates RARβ and RARγ, as does adapalene. Tazarotene is licensed for the treatment of acne in the USA but not currently in the UK or Italy.

Isotretinoin. Topical isotretinoin is an alternative preparation available as a 0.05% gel in the UK and Italy but not currently available in the USA. This novel retinoid has been shown to be less irritant than older retinoid preparations such as tretinoin.

Salicylic, α-hydroxy and azelaic acids

Salicylic acid is keratolytic and an irritant which may promote the resolution of inflammatory lesions through its drying effect. Salicylic acid has mild comedolytic activity. It is available in a maximum concentration of 2% in over-the-counter preparations such as soaps, cleansers and gel preparations. Some salicylic acid products are tinted to help camouflage acne lesions. Products containing salicylic acid in combination with benzoyl peroxide or sulfur are also available.

Alpha-hydroxy acids are fruit acids, such as lactic acid, glycolic acid and citric acid. They are available in a variety of cosmetic preparations, including cleansers, toners, moisturizers and chemical peels. Alpha-hydroxy acids are thought to reverse the altered keratinization of follicles affected by acne and also improve the appearance of the skin by promoting desquamation of the stratum corneum. The effectiveness of α-hydroxy acids in acne, however, has not yet been demonstrated in controlled clinical trials.

Azelaic acid is a naturally occurring dicarboxylic acid found in cereal grains. It is available as a topical cream which has been shown to be effective in inflammatory and comedonal acne. By inhibiting the growth of *P. acnes*, azelaic acid reduces inflammatory acne. It also reverses the altered keratinization of follicles seen in acne and thus demonstrates comedolytic activity. The activity of azelaic acid against inflammatory lesions may be greater than its activity against comedones. Azelaic acid is reported to have fewer local side effects than topical retinoids.

Topical antibiotics

Topical antibiotics such as erythromycin, clindamycin, and sodium sulfacetamide inhibit the growth of *P. acnes* and reduce inflammatory lesions. Products containing these antibiotics are often applied twice daily and are generally well tolerated. Topical antibiotics such as erythromycin and clindamycin come in a variety of vehicles and packaging. Vehicles include creams, lotions, ointments, gels and solutions. Solutions are available in dab-on applicators and pads which are packaged either individually or in bulk. The choice of vehicle or packaging depends on the patient's complexion and preference. Many teenagers enjoy the convenience of the pad preparations. Sodium sulfacetamide is a sulfonamide which is thought to inhibit the growth of *P. acnes* through competitive antagonism of para-aminobenzoic acid, an essential requirement for bacterial growth. Sodium sulfacetamide (10%) is available combined with sulfur (5%) in a prescription lotion either with or without tint. Topical tetracycline is available in the UK and Italy.

Combination products

Topical erythromycin has been combined with benzoyl peroxide and also with zinc in an effort to enhance its efficacy in acne. These products are generally applied twice daily. Some erythromycin / benzoyl peroxide combinations require refrigeration. Studies have shown that in addition to their efficacy in reducing acne lesions, use of these products may decrease the proliferation of resistant strains of *P. acnes*. Topical isotretinoin is available in combination with erythromycin in the UK and Italy. One recent study has demonstrated that the topical combination containing benzoyl peroxide and clindamycin produced good efficacy. The combination products are very effective in mild-to-early-moderate acne. They offer convenience of use, particularly for the teenage patient who may be less willing to adhere to regimens using different topical medications. Combining products with a synergistic effect can also help to reduce side effects.

Side effects of topical therapy

Most topical acne treatments, including salicylic acid, benzoyl peroxide and topical retinoids, will cause some degree of erythema, dryness and scaling of the skin. As a peroxide, benzoyl peroxide can bleach clothing or bedding, particularly when it is applied to the chest or back. This problem can be circumvented by recommending that the medication be used at bedtime and that treated areas be covered with an old shirt. Contact dermatitis to benzoyl peroxide has rarely been reported but should be considered if treated areas develop an eczematous dermatitis. Use of topical antibiotics may also be associated with local irritation, but this tends to occur less often than with other topical agents. The local side effects of topical retinoids include erythema, scaling, desquamation, burning or stinging, pruritus and increased susceptibility to sunburn. Most patients will develop tolerance to the local side effects of topical retinoids within 3–4 weeks. If patients are unable to tolerate daily application of a topical retinoid, an alternate day or an every-third-day regimen can be followed until tolerance develops. In this case, the goal is to accustom the patient's skin gradually to the medication so that daily application will eventually be possible. Topical retinoids may also provoke an acne flare; this is less evident with the novel preparations isotretinoin and adapalene.

Because of their teratogenic potential, use of topical retinoids in pregnancy is not recommended. Fortunately, studies have shown that the risk of birth defects from use of topical tretinoin is small. Pharmacokinetic studies have shown that serum retinoid levels may be influenced more by diet than by facial application of topical tretinoin for acne. Epidemiological studies have failed to demonstrate an increased risk of birth defects in infants whose mothers used topical retinoids on the face during the first trimester of pregnancy. There have, however, been isolated case reports of birth defects in infants whose mothers used topical tretinoin during pregnancy. For this reason, it is recommended that a woman cease using topical retinoids if she is, or is trying to become, pregnant.

P. acnes resistance is an emerging problem and is believed to be driven by antibiotic usage, particularly of topical antibiotics. It is important to bear this in mind when prescribing antibiotics, because the relevance of *P. acnes* resistance in clinical outcomes of acne has been demonstrated. Using benzoyl peroxide preparations concurrently with or between antibiotic courses will be effective, at the site of application, against antibiotic-resistant *P. acnes* strains and will prevent the development of further resistant strains.

Management of side effects

Excessive dryness of the skin is one of the main reasons why patients discontinue treatment. Thus, recommendations regarding effective ways of managing facial dryness should be an integral part of any acne treatment plan. Many patients are reluctant to use facial moisturizers because they are concerned that moisturizers might worsen their acne. Nowadays most moisturizers from reputable companies are tested for comedogenicity in clinical trials and are labeled 'noncomedogenic'. Moisturizers are available as creams, lotions and ointments. Most patients prefer to use lotions because they are easy to apply and do not feel greasy. Lotions containing sunscreens should be recommended, particularly in patients using topical retinoids. For recalcitrant dry areas, a heavier cream may be needed. Ointments should be avoided as they are more comedogenic. The regular use of moisturizers is especially important for patients receiving topical acne therapy.

The use of sunscreens is also important. Any facial irritation that may occur as a result of topical acne medications can be exacerbated by the sun. In addition a number of topical preparations make patients more photosensitive. Thus, regular use of a sunscreen or a moisturizer containing a sunscreen is recommended.

If irritation remains a problem despite adequate use of moisturizers, the treatment regimen can be temporarily altered. For example, topical retinoids could be used every other day or every third day until tolerance is obtained, or the duration of application could be gradually increased until tolerated. The goal will then be to increase gradually the frequency of application until the patient can tolerate daily application.

Guidelines for managing acne with topical therapy

With the exception of early comedonal acne in prepubertal children, it is rare for a patient to present with a single type of acne lesion. For this reason, combination therapy is a mainstay of acne treatment. Different topical therapies may be alternated morning and evening, or formulations containing a stable combination of products (see page 41) may be prescribed. Therapeutic agents should be chosen to match the type and severity of lesions observed in each individual patient. Comedonal acne with a mild inflammatory component can be managed with novel topical retinoids as first-line therapy. If this fails and the extent of the inflammatory lesions increases, the addition of topical antibiotics and/or benzoyl peroxide should be considered. As the inflammatory component of acne increases, oral antibiotics (systemic therapy) should be used in place of topical antibiotics. In general the addition of a topical antibiotic to a regimen containing oral antibiotics offers no additional benefit; furthermore, if based on a different chemical group, it may lead to the development of multiple-antibiotic-resistant strains of bacteria. Microcomedones are the precursor lesions of both inflammatory and non-inflammatory acne; therefore a topical therapy aimed at reducing microcomedones may be useful as maintenance therapy. The inclusion of benzoyl peroxide in any acne therapeutic regimen containing antibiotics is beneficial because this agent has potent bactericidal activity against both antibiotic-resistant and -sensitive *P. acnes* and can retard the development of antibiotic-resistant strains at the site of application.

Key points – topical therapy

- Topical therapy should be directed at the lesion type, extent and severity of acne.
- Topical therapy should be selected to enable compliance. Realistic expectations of therapy should be explained.
- Combining therapies or using manufacturer-combined therapies improves efficacy by directing treatment more specifically.
- Topical antibiotics predispose patients to develop antibiotic-resistant strains of *Propionibacterium acnes*.
- Benzoyl peroxide preparations can reduce and prevent the development of antibiotic-resistant strains of *P. acnes* at the site of application.
- The novel topical retinoids are less irritant and produce less acne flare than older topical retinoids.

Key references

Bernard BA. Adapalene, a new chemical entity with retinoid activity. *Skin Pharmacol* 1993; 6(suppl):61–9.

Bershad S, Singer GK, Parente JE et al. Successful treatment of acne vulgaris using a new method. *Arch Dermatol* 2002;138:481–9.

Bojard R, Eady E, Jones C. Inhibition of erythromycin-resistant propioni-bacteria on the skin of acne patients by topical erythromycin with and without zinc. *Br J Dermatol* 1994;130:329–36.

Eady AE, Cove JH, Layton AM. Is antibiotic resistance in cutaneous propionibacteria clinically relevant? *Am J Clin Dermatol* 2003;4:813–31.

Fulton J, Farzad-Bakshandeh A, Bradley S. Studies on the mechanism of action of topical benzoyl peroxide and vitamin A acid in acne vulgaris. *J Cutan Pathol* 1974;1:191–200.

Gollnick H, Krautheim A. Topical treatment in acne: current status and future aspects. *Dermatology* 2003;206:29–36.

Gollnick H, Graupe K. Azelaic acid for the treatment of acne: comparative trials. *J Dermatol Treat* 1989;1:27–30.

Gollnick H, Schramm M. Topical drug treatment in acne. *Dermatology* 1998;196:119–25.

Hughes BR, Norris H, Cunliffe WJ. A double blind evaluation of topical isotretinoin 0.05%, benzoyl peroxide gel 5% and placebo in patients with acne. *Clin Exp Dermatol* 1992; 17:165–8.

Kaminsky A. Less common methods to treat acne. *Dermatology* 2003;206:68–73.

Leyden JJ. A review of the use of combination therapies for the treatment of acne vulgaris. *J Am Acad Dermatol* 2003; 49 (suppl 3):S200–10.

Lucky AW, Cullen SI, Jarrat MT. Comparative efficacy and safety of two 0.025% tretinoin gels: results from a multicenter, double-blind, parallel study. *J Am Acad Dermatol* 1998;38:817–23.

Ross J, Snelling AM, Carnegie E et al. Antibiotic-resistant acne: lessons from Europe. *Br J Dermatol* 2003; 148:467–78.

Shalita AR. A multicenter double blind controlled study of the combination of erythromycin/benzoyl peroxide, erythromycin alone and benzoyl peroxide alone in the treatment of acne vulgaris. *Cutis* 1992;49:1–4.

Soffman MS, Shalita AR. Topical antibiotic treatment of acne. In: Marks R, Plewig G, eds. *Acne and Related Disorders*. London: Martin Dunitz, 1989:159–64.

Webster G. Topical tretinoin in acne therapy. *J Am Acad Dermatol* 1998;39(2 part 3):338–44.

Wolf JE. An update on recent clinical trials examining adapalene and acne. *J Eur Acad Dermatol Venereol* 2001;15(suppl):23–9.

Effective systemic therapies for acne include antibiotics, hormonal therapies for women, and isotretinoin.

Systemic antibiotics

Table 6.1 summarizes the range of oral antibiotic therapy available for acne, and appropriate dosage. Systemic antibiotics such as erythromycin and oxytetracycline, or the derivatives doxycycline, lymecycline and minocycline, are most often used for moderate-to-severe inflammatory acne not responding to topical combinations. The primary mechanism of action of these agents in acne treatment is suppression of the growth of *P. acnes*, thereby reducing inflammatory factors. Many of these antibiotics also possess intrinsic anti-inflammatory activity.

Erythromycin. Oral erythromycin is comparable to oxytetracycline in its therapeutic effect on acne, although resistance of *P. acnes* to erythromycin is much more common. Generally, erythromycin is given in doses of 500 mg twice daily.

Oxytetracycline, doxycycline, lymecycline and minocycline. Oxytetracycline and its derivatives are the most commonly used oral medications for acne vulgaris. Tetracycline hydrochloride is known to penetrate sebocytes and keratinocytes to reach the follicular canal. An initial starting dose is 500 mg twice daily. Second-generation tetracyclines, such as lymecycline, doxycycline and minocycline, show improved absorption and hence more rapid efficacy. Doxycycline is a lipophilic tetracycline derivative with demonstrated efficacy in the treatment of inflammatory acne. As for oxytetracycline, resistance of *P. acnes* to doxycycline has been reported. Doxycycline can be given in doses of 100–200 mg daily; recently, a dose of 50 mg daily has been used. Minocycline, also a lipophilic derivative of tetracycline, achieves excellent penetration into the follicular canal. It is often effective in

TABLE 6.1

Oral antibiotics available for acne

Drug/dose	Comments regarding usage	Incidence of P. acnes resistance	Adverse effects	
			Common	Rare
Oxytetracycline/ tetracycline 500 mg twice daily	Inexpensive: take 30 minutes before food and not with milk	Moderate	GI upset, including nausea, diarrhea, dysphagia, esophageal irritation	Allergic rashes, photosensitivity, hepatotoxicity
Erythromycin 500 mg twice daily	Inexpensive	High	GI upset, including nausea, diarrhea, abdominal discomfort	Allergic rashes, cholestatic jaundice
Minocycline 100–200 mg daily	Expensive	Low (in 1999) but increasing	GI upset less common than with (oxy)tetracycline	Pigmentary changes, BIH, autoimmune hepatitis
Doxycycline 100–200 mg daily	Inexpensive	Moderate	As (oxy)tetracycline	Photosensitivity (dose dependent)
Lymecycline 300–600 mg daily	Moderately expensive	Moderate	As (oxy)tetracycline	As (oxy)tetracycline
Trimethoprim 200–300 mg twice daily	Inexpensive	Low (in 1999)	GI upset including nausea and vomiting, rashes	Photosensitivity, very rarely agranulocytosis

The use of 'megadose' (i.e. high-dose) antibiotics may be required for patients with greasy skin (i.e. with a high sebum excretion rate), high body mass (probably because of high blood volume rather than weight), and/or who are colonized by P. acnes with reduced sensitivity
BIH, benign intracranial hypertension

cases of acne that have not responded to treatment with other oral antibiotics. It has potent anti-inflammatory properties and has been shown to be more effective than oxytetracycline. There are fewer reports of resistance of *P. acnes* to minocycline compared with tetracycline and doxycycline; however, this is changing. Reduced response to minocycline should be suspected in patients from whom isolates are tetracycline resistant, because minocycline minimum inhibitory concentrations are raised for such isolates. If patients have not responded after 6–8 weeks of minocycline, 200 mg daily, referral for isotretinoin therapy should be considered. Lymecycline, 300–600 mg daily, is also available for acne. Studies have demonstrated that it is as effective as oral minocycline and has a lower side-effect profile. Lymecycline breaks down into tetracycline, lysine and formaldehyde in the gastrointestinal tract. The incidence of *P. acnes* resistance therefore mirrors that of tetracycline.

Trimethoprim is an alternative systemic antibiotic that can be used as third-line therapy for the treatment of acne at a dose of 200–300 mg twice daily. Adverse effects include skin rashes and, very rarely, agranulocytosis.

Optimizing antibiotic therapy. Principles for the optimum use of oral antibiotics are discussed on page 57.

Hormonal therapy

It is important to note that hormonal therapy can be very effective in females with acne whether or not their serum androgens are abnormal. Although women with acne may have higher serum androgens than those without acne, these levels are often still within the normal range. Hormonal therapies seem to work best in women with persistent inflammatory papules and nodules that commonly involve the lower face and neck. Often, these women report that their acne flares prior to their menstrual periods and consists of a few tender deep-seated inflammatory papules and nodules. The skin may or may not be oily. Comedones are often present on the forehead and chin. These patients often note little improvement in their acne despite multiple courses of various antibiotics.

In such cases, oral antibiotics can be discontinued and therapy with oral contraceptives initiated, because they block both the ovarian and adrenal production of androgens. In addition, use of oral contraceptives is recommended if treatment with spironolactone is anticipated, since feminization of the male fetus will occur if pregnancy ensues. Because of the potential risks associated with oral contraceptive use and the need for breast and pelvic examinations, consultation with a gynecologist is recommended. A preparation containing a progestin with low androgenic activity such as norgestimate or ethinyl estradiol / cyproterone acetate is appropriate. If the patient's acne has not improved significantly after three to six cycles, spironolactone can be added.

Oral contraceptives

Oral estrogen/progestin. Estrogens are most commonly used to treat acne in combination with a progestin in order to avoid the risk of endometrial cancer associated with unopposed estrogens. The beneficial effects of oral contraceptives on acne have been noted for many years. Oral contraceptives are thought to exert their antiacne effect by decreasing the level of circulating androgens. Specifically, they have been shown to increase sex-hormone-binding globulin and decrease free testosterone in healthy women. In addition, the estrogen component may decrease the production of ovarian androgens by suppressing the secretion of pituitary gonadotropins. Unfortunately, many progestins also have intrinsic androgenic activity which can aggravate acne. Of the second-generation progestins, ethynodiol diacetate, norethindrone and levonorgestrel had the lowest androgenic activity. The third-generation progestins – desogestrel, norgestimate and gestodene – have the lowest intrinsic androgenic activity. Although available in Europe, gestodene is not currently available in the USA.

Norgestimate–ethinyl estradiol (Ortho TriCyclen). This triphasic, combination oral contraceptive is the first low-dose oral contraceptive to receive approval from the Food and Drug Administration (FDA) for the treatment of acne in the USA. The efficacy of the norgestimate–ethinyl estradiol combination in the treatment of acne was demonstrated in two 6-month, randomized, placebo-controlled trials, each of which enrolled approximately 250 women with moderate acne. In each study, the active group was significantly better than the placebo group for all primary efficacy measures: inflammatory lesions, total lesions, and investigator's global assessment. No significant adverse effects were reported in these trials.

Cyproterone acetate (CPA) is a progestational antiandrogen that blocks the androgen receptor. It is available in Europe and Canada, but not in the USA. It is of use in patients with acne resistant to other therapies and reduces sebum production. In addition it may have a direct effect on comedogenesis, which is known to be androgen mediated. CPA, 2 mg, is combined with ethinyl estradiol, 35 µg, in an oral contraceptive formulation, co-cyprindiol (Dianette), that is widely used in Europe for the treatment of acne. Co-cyprindiol is the treatment of choice in patients who need oral therapy and who are sexually active and need a contraceptive pill, or in those patients who need hormonal therapy to regulate disorganized periods.

CPA alone has also been used to treat acne. Overall improvement in 75–90% of patients treated with CPA, 50–100 mg daily, with or without ethinyl estradiol, 35–50 µg, has been reported.

Levonorgestrel–ethinyl estradiol. Two large, 6-month, placebo-controlled trials examined ethinyl estradiol–levonorgestrel, 20+100 µg (Alesse), in the treatment of acne. In each study, the oral contraceptive demonstrated significantly greater reduction in acne lesion counts and improvement in global assessment scores compared to placebo.

Norethindrone acetate–ethinyl estradiol (Estrostep). Two large placebo-controlled studies, involving a total of 593 women with moderate acne, found improvement in inflammatory lesions, total lesions, global assessment and quality of life in women who were treated for 6 months with a triphasic oral contraceptive which contains doses of 20 to 35 mg of ethinyl estradiol in combination with 1.0 mg norethindrone acetate. This oral contraceptive has been approved in the USA for the treatment of acne.

Drospirenone is a novel progestin derived from 17α-spironolactone. It possesses antiandrogenic and antimineralocorticoid activity, which can be of benefit in androgenic conditions, such as acne and hirsutism, and in the estrogen-related fluid retention associated with some oral contraceptives. A recent study of 128 women with mild-to-moderate acne compared the efficacy of ethinyl estradiol, 30 µg–drospirenone (Yasmin) and ethinyl estradiol, 35 µg–cyproterone acetate (Diane-35) in the treatment of acne for 9 cycles. The treatments produced comparable reductions of approximately 60% in inflammatory lesion count. Both treatments also reduced sebum production and yielded comparable increases in sex-hormone-binding globulin.

Spironolactone functions both as an androgen-receptor blocker and inhibitor of 5α-reductase. In doses of 50–100 mg twice daily, it has been shown to reduce sebum production and improve acne. Lower doses can also be effective in acne. It is recommended that treatment be initiated with a low dose such as 25–50 mg twice daily. The dose can be increased if the patient is not experiencing significant breast tenderness or headache. Effective maintenance doses are in the range of 25–200 mg per day. Response in acne may take up to 3 months, as with other hormonal therapies.

Systemic retinoids

Oral isotretinoin (13-*cis*-retinoic acid) is a specialist-only drug in most countries and is prescribed:

- for patients with severe acne
- for patients in whom adequate oral and topical therapy has failed
- in the presence of significant physical or psychological scarring.

Isotretinoin is a retinoid (a vitamin A derivative) with the unique ability to reduce the size and secretion of sebaceous glands. Oral isotretinoin is the most effective agent available for severe inflammatory acne or nodulocystic acne. It is the only drug that affects all four pathogenic factors implicated in the etiology of acne. Isotretinoin produces an 80% reduction in sebum excretion, reduces comedogenesis, and lowers ductal and surface *P. acnes* within 4–8 weeks of the start of treatment. It also demonstrates anti-inflammatory activity.

Since its inception, the use of oral isotretinoin treatment has been responsible for a dramatic improvement in the appearance and psychological wellbeing of numerous individuals affected by cystic acne. The dose usually depends on factors such as age, sex and body weight of the patient. At the end of an adequate course, acne will have cleared in a large proportion of patients. Complete cure is thought to be effected in 50–70% of cases; however, as the remit for oral isotretinoin has broadened over the last decade, there are no accurate figures. What is certain is that a course of oral isotretinoin alters the state of the skin, and so many treatments that were not helpful before isotretinoin administration become efficacious thereafter. A small minority of patients will require a further course of oral isotretinoin.

The use of oral isotretinoin is limited by its side-effect profile (see pages 55–6).

Side effects of oral therapy

Antibiotics. Oral antibiotics are occasionally associated with gastrointestinal upsets such as nausea, colic and diarrhea (Table 6.1). Vaginal candidiasis may be a problem in sexually active females, and treatment of both partners is necessary to control this problem adequately. Other side effects are rare. An interaction of oral contraceptives and long-term antibiotics, making the oral contraceptive less effective, has been reported as a possibility and should be discussed with the patient. However, a recent review by Archer and Archer suggested that available laboratory and pharmacokinetic data do not support this hypothesis. Patients should, however, be warned about possible reduced effect if vomiting or diarrhea occur. An unusual side effect of long-term antibiotics is pseudomembranous colitis, but in the authors' experience this is exceedingly rare.

Erythromycin. The most common adverse effect associated with erythromycin is gastrointestinal irritation. This may be alleviated to some degree by taking the drug with food or milk, but this is likely to reduce absorption of the drug.

Oxytetracycline/doxycycline. Side effects of tetracyclines are well-known and include gastrointestinal upset, vaginal yeast infection, and possible decreased efficacy of oral contraceptives. Doxycycline is associated with a dose-dependent light-sensitive rash. Patients need to be warned about this and given adequate advice about using a sunscreen. The use of tetracyclines as a class is not recommended in patients under 9 years of age in the USA and under 12 years of age in the UK. Tetracyclines should not be used in pregnant patients, to avoid the risks of tooth discoloration and bone growth retardation in the fetus.

Minocycline is one of the most effective antibiotics in the treatment of acne. Unlike the less lipophilic tetracyclines, minocycline is associated with vestibular side effects such as headache, dizziness, ataxia and drowsiness. In view of the potential risks of minocycline, including pseudotumor cerebri, pigmentation of skin, sclera and bone, autoimmune hepatitis, serum-sickness-like reactions and drug-induced lupus, it is important to counsel patients to report any symptoms associated with their therapy. The physician should perform a review of symptoms at follow-up visits to encompass these potential side effects in addition to physical examination of the skin, sclera and oral cavity for signs of pigment deposition which may occur in patients receiving high doses for prolonged periods of time. The pigmentation associated with the use of minocycline occurs in acne scars (Figure 6.1) and other scars and much more rarely in the mucosae, sclera and nails. The skin pigmentation may last for many months after therapy is stopped.

As a result of its lipophilicity, minocycline penetrates the blood–brain barrier, where it may precipitate pseudotumor cerebri syndrome, presenting as headaches, dizziness and blurred vision. This is a rare side effect of high-dose minocycline and is reversible if therapy is promptly stopped. In a retrospective study conducted in an academic neuro-ophthalmic referral center, 12 cases of pseudotumor cerebri syndrome associated with minocycline therapy were reviewed. These patients were receiving minocycline, 50–200 mg daily, for the treatment of acne. The duration of treatment ranged from less than 1 week to 1 year. The most common symptoms were headache (75%), transient visual disturbances (41%), diplopia (41%), pulsatile tinnitus (17%) and nausea and vomiting (25%). Nine (75%) of the 12 patients developed symptoms of pseudotumor cerebri syndrome within 8 weeks of starting therapy. Two patients developed symptoms after 1 year. One patient was asymptomatic, and papilledema was found on routine eye examination. All but one patient were treated with acetazolamide to reduce the intracranial pressure. After 1 year of

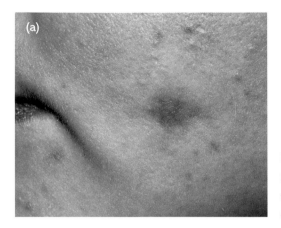

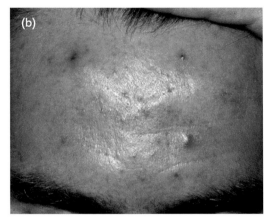

Figure 6.1 Minocycline pigmentation: (a) subtle, gray/blue pigmentation at site of previous acne on cheek; (b) dark gray deposits on forehead, like 'lead pencil' marks.

follow-up, no recurrences were noted after the discontinuation of minocycline, but 3 of the 12 subjects had substantial residual visual field loss.

Very rare side effects of minocycline include a serum-sickness-like illness (urticaria vasculitis, arthritis and fever). This usually occurs within 3 months; after 10–12 months of therapy, hepatitis associated with a lupus-like syndrome may also occur very rarely. In all these patients minocycline should be discontinued. With vigilance on the part of the physician, minocycline can be used safely and effectively in the treatment of acne. It is advisable to monitor liver function and autoantibodies in patients receiving minocycline for periods greater than 6 months.

Hormonal therapy

Oral contraceptives. All oral contraceptives, including those used to treat acne, have similar side effects.

The most common adverse effects associated with oral contraceptives as a class are nausea, vomiting, breakthrough bleeding, weight gain and breast tenderness. Rare but serious adverse effects include hypertension, thrombophlebitis and pulmonary embolism.

There is controversy in the literature as to whether there is an increased risk of venous thromboembolism associated with oral contraceptives containing desogestrel and gestodene. The risk of myocardial infarction, however, may be lower in women using these oral contraceptives than in those using one containing a second-generation progestin.

Spironolactone. The side effects are dose-related and include potential hyperkalemia, irregular menstrual periods, breast tenderness, headache and fatigue. Hyperkalemia is rare in young, healthy patients. Although breast tumors have been reported in rodent models treated with spironolactone, the drug has not been directly linked to the development of cancer in humans. As this medication is an antiandrogen, there is a risk of feminization of a male fetus if it is taken by a pregnant woman.

Isotretinoin is a known teratogen. Pregnancy is completely contraindicated. Given this, a negative pregnancy test must be obtained from female patients of childbearing potential prior to initiation of therapy, and education regarding the need for adequate contraception must be given. Pregnancy testing is carried out before initiating therapy and monthly thereafter in the USA; it is carried out before initiating therapy in the UK. Adequate contraception should be used for 1 month before, during and for 6 weeks after stopping therapy.

Other adverse effects of isotretinoin include mucocutaneous problems, i.e. cheilitis, epistaxis, dry skin, and ocular and vaginal dryness. Arthralgia, secondary skin infection with *Staphylococcus aureus*, and, rarely, pseudotumor cerebri and skeletal hyperostosis have also been reported. The mucocutaneous symptoms occur in virtually all

55

patients, particularly dry lips, dry skin and occasionally dry eyes. Musculoskeletal side effects are quite common, in up to 20% of subjects, including low-grade muscle and joint pain.

Elevations of serum triglycerides or liver enzymes may occur, but are not usually clinically significant. Headaches also occasionally occur. Mood swings have been reported in patients taking isotretinoin. More recently the FDA and the UK Medicines Control Agency (MCA) have issued a warning that depression may be an uncommon idiosyncratic and unpredictable adverse effect associated with systemic isotretinoin therapy. This must be discussed with the patient and, if relevant, close relatives. It is suggested that baseline liver function tests and fasting lipid profile be obtained, with follow-up monitoring ranging from every 4–8 weeks to less frequently if baseline values are normal.

Because of this complex side-effect profile, successful use of isotretinoin in the treatment of acne requires careful patient selection and education, and appropriate monitoring and follow-up on the part of an experienced dermatologist. Patients receiving oral isotretinoin should be given immediate access to the dermatologist if there is any problem with therapy or a failure to respond adequately to the drug.

Management of side effects

Antibiotics. The lower abdominal symptoms can often be controlled by the judicious use of loperamide taken once/twice daily if colic or diarrhea is a problem. The current recommendation from the UK Royal College of General Practitioners is that physical methods of contraception should be used during the first month of co-prescribing.

Minocycline pigmentation can be improved by using a Q-switched ruby laser.

Spironolactone. Risk to a fetus and the symptoms of irregular menstrual bleeding can be alleviated by combining treatment with an oral contraceptive. Side effects can be minimized if therapy is initiated with a low dose (25–50 mg daily).

Isotretinoin. The common side effects of isotretinoin such as xerosis of the skin, dry eyes and musculoskeletal symptoms are usually well controlled by dose adjustment and by simple measures such as moisturizers, non-steroidal anti-inflammatory drugs and paracetamol. The regular use of moisturizers is especially important for patients receiving isotretinoin, who are at risk of developing fissuring of the skin with secondary infection. Use of moisturizers and lip balm that contain sunscreens will help prevent these complications. Artificial tears can be used to alleviate the problem of dry eyes.

In rare cases, patients may experience hypertriglyceridemia that persists even with dose adjustment. Initially these patients should modify their diet to reduce their intake of fatty foods. Rarely, concomitant therapy with a drug such as gemfibrizol may be required to manage the hypertriglyceridemia.

If patients experience any significant change in mood, they are advised to stop their therapy and seek the advice of their dermatologist.

Guidelines for managing acne with oral therapy

The choice of treatment should depend on the acne lesions and severity as well as the presence of scarring and/or psychological disability.

Antibiotics. Second-generation tetracycline antibiotics should now probably be the systemic treatment of choice for those patients who can tolerate them. These include lymecycline, 300 mg twice daily, and doxycycline or minocycline, 100–200 mg daily. Second-generation tetracyclines are absorbed more rapidly, are more rapidly efficacious and achieve better compliance than first-generation tetracyclines. Minocycline is thought to be associated with the lowest incidence of antibiotic *P. acnes* resistance but, as with topical antibiotics, development of resistance of *P. acnes* to oral tetracyclines is a potential problem. This should be suspected if a patient's acne fails to respond or improves then worsens after several months of treatment with tetracycline. In such cases, an alternative agent should be chosen. Erythromycin is now used less frequently because of increasing bacterial resistance. It is the drug of choice in women who 'may become' pregnant. The third-line treatment is oral trimethoprim, 200–300 mg twice daily.

Antibiotics have often been given for prolonged periods: up to 6–12 months, with repeat courses over months or years. Research has demonstrated that problems of antibiotic-resistant *P. acnes* have resulted on an international scale. The emergence of resistance has raised the issue of the need for antibiotic prescribing policies and the need to consider the use of non-antibiotic preparations wherever possible. Current thinking is that antibiotics should be administered for as short a duration as possible, and that combining them initially with topical retinoids will enhance efficacy. If a course longer than 12 weeks is required, anti-resistance agents, for example benzoyl peroxide, should be used concurrently. Combining non-antibiotic and antibiotic therapies results in more rapid efficacy, and this in turn may reduce the antibiotic exposure time. The same antibiotic should be used again if it previously produced a good clinical response. If both topical and oral antibiotics are required, they should be of the same chemical group to prevent development of multiple strains of resistant *P. acnes*. Principles for the optimal use of oral antibiotics are summarized in Table 6.2.

Orally administered tetracyclines, erythromycin and trimethoprim are effective in the management of moderate-to-severe acne. However, as systemic agents, they are associated with more significant and more diverse side-effect profiles than many topical agents. These agents are

TABLE 6.2

Optimizing oral antibiotic therapy

- Use only in moderate to severe acne
- Avoid using as monotherapy
- Combining with topical retinoids provides more rapid efficacy
- Combining with benzoyl peroxide reduces likelihood of resistance
- Duration of use:
    - minimum 6 weeks
    - maximum 12 weeks
- If duration > 12 weeks, use anti-resistance agents concurrently
- Avoid switching antibiotics
- Encourage compliance
- Advise on potential side effects

increasingly associated with the development of resistance by *P. acnes*. For these reasons, careful patient selection and management are required when the addition of systemic antibiotics to an antiacne regimen is under consideration.

The expected response of acne to systemic antibiotic therapy is shown in Figure 6.2. Note that there is little improvement in the first month, but by 8 months there should be 80% improvement. If after 3 months there is no or little improvement, alternative therapy to that already given should be considered.

Hormonal therapy. In Europe, Dianette is the treatment of choice in patients with moderate acne who need oral therapy and who are sexually active and need a contraceptive pill, or in those patients who need hormonal therapy to regulate disorganized menstrual periods. In the USA, the FDA-approved Ortho TriCyclen is the treatment of choice in patients fitting this description. The popularity of the oral contraceptive containing drospirenone (Yasmin) is increasing in both areas, and studies of its use in acne are under way. As with regimens

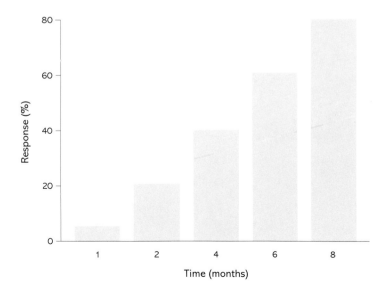

Figure 6.2 Expected response to systemic antibiotic therapy.

containing oral antibiotics, if the patient has comedones in addition to inflammatory lesions, agents such as topical retinoids should be added to the antiacne regimen.

Isotretinoin. Indications for the use of oral isotretinoin, discussed on page 51, are listed in Table 6.3. There are a variety of approaches to therapy with this drug. In Europe, patients are generally treated with 0.5 mg/kg/day until a total dose of 120–150 mg/kg has been attained. In the USA, therapy may be initiated with 0.5 mg/kg/day for the first month and then the dose may be increased to 1.0 mg/kg/day for a total of 20 weeks of therapy. It is especially important that therapy be initiated at the lower dose in patients whose severe acne is highly inflammatory, particularly if it involves the chest and back in addition to the face. Young men with this type of acne are at a particular risk of developing a severe flare of their inflammatory or cystic acne. In some cases, exuberant lesions similar to pyogenic granulomas may develop. It is strongly recommended that patients with severe inflammatory cystic acne who are at risk of these complications be referred to the dermatologist for treatment with isotretinoin and possibly a concomitant course of oral corticosteroids.

Dosage regimens for isotretinoin are being re-evaluated, as many of the previous recommendations are based on regimens used for severe or non-responding acne. The remit for the use of oral isotretinoin has expanded over the last few years.

TABLE 6.3

Indications for systemic isotretinoin

- Severe nodular inflammatory acne
- Moderate acne unresponsive to conventional therapy
- Moderate acne relapsing after conventional therapy
- Development of acne scarring
- Psychological disability related to acne or scarring
- Unusual variants of acne

Key points – oral therapy

• Systemic antibiotics remain useful therapy for inflammatory acne.

• Antibiotic-resistant *Propionibacterium acnes* constitutes an emerging problem, and prescribing should take this important factor into account.

• Antiandrogen hormonal therapy may be helpful in female patients.

• Oral isotretinoin should be considered in patients with severe, scarring acne and those who have relapsed or are not responding to conventional therapy.

• Oral isotretinoin is teratogenic, and careful monitoring is mandatory.

• Oral isotretinoin has been linked to depression and suicide, and patients should be carefully counseled about the risks.

Key references

Altman RS, Altman LJ, Altman JS. A proposed set of new guidelines for routine blood tests during isotretinoin therapy for acne vulgaris. *Dermatology* 2002;204:232–5.

Archer JS, Archer DF. Oral contraceptive efficacy and antibiotic interaction: a myth debunked. *J Am Acad Dermatol* 2002;46:917–23.

Beylot C, Doutre MS, Beylot-Barry M. Oral contraceptives and cyproterone acetate in female acne treatment. *Dermatology* 1998;196:148–52.

Bickers DR, Saurat JH. Isotretinoin: a state of the art conference. *J Am Acad Dermatol* 2001;45:S125–8.

Bottomley WW, Cunliffe WJ. Oral trimethoprim as a third line antibiotic in the management of acne vulgaris. *Dermatology* 1993;187:193–6.

Cunliffe WJ, Meynadier J, Alirezai M et al. Is combined oral and topical therapy better than oral therapy alone in patients with moderate to moderately severe acne vulgaris? A comparison of the efficacy and safety of lymecycline plus adapalene gel 0.1% versus lymecycline plus gel vehicle. *J Am Acad Dermatol* 2003;49(suppl 3):S218–26.

Garner SE, Eady EA, Popescu C et al. Minocycline for acne vulgaris: efficacy and safety. *Cochrane Database Syst Rev* 2002;2: CD 002086.

Gollnick H, Cunliffe W, Berson D et al. Management of acne. A report from a global alliance to improve outcomes in acne. *J Am Acad Dermatol* 2003;49(suppl 1):S1–37.

Leyden J. Current issues in antimicrobial therapy for the treatment of acne. *J Eur Acad Dermatol Venereol* 2001;15 (suppl 3):51–5.

Leyden J, Powala C, Ashley R. Effects of subantimicrobial-dose doxycycline in the treatment of moderate acne. *Arch Dermatol* 2003;139:459–64.

Leyden J, Shalita A, Hordinsky M. et al. Efficacy of a low-dose oral contraceptive containing 20 mg of ethinyl estradiol and 100 µg of levonorgestrel for the treatment of moderate acne: A randomized, placebo-controlled trial. *J Am Acad Dermatol* 2002;47:399–409.

Maloney M, Arbit DI, Flack M et al. Use of a low-dose oral contraceptive containing norethindrone acetate and ethinyl estradiol in the treatment of moderate acne vulgaris. *Clin J Womens Health* 2001;1:124–31.

McLane J. Analysis of common side effects of isotretinoin. *J Am Acad Dermatol* 2001;45:S188–94.

Meynadier J, Alizerai M. Systemic antibiotic for acne. *Dermatology* 1998;196:135–9.

Nau H. Teratogenicity of isotretinoin revisited: species variations and the role of all-trans-retinoic acid. *J Am Acad Dermatol* 2001;45:S183-7.

Shaw JC. Low-dose adjunctive spironolactone in the treatment of acne in women: a retrospective analysis of 83 consecutively treated patients. *J Am Acad Dermatol* 2000;43:498–502.

Schollhammer M, Alirezai M. Etude comparative de la lymecycline (Tetralysal), de la minocycline (Mynocin), et de la doxycycline (Tolexine) dans le traitement de l'acne vulgaire. *Réal Thér Derm Vénéréol* 1994;42:24–6.

Stoll S, Shalita AR, Webster GF et al. The effect of menstrual cycle on acne. *J Am Acad Dermatol* 2001;45: 957–60.

Thiboutot D, Archer D, Lemay A et al. A randomized, controlled trial of a low-dose contraceptive containing 20 µg of ethinylestradiol and 100 µg of levonorgestrel for acne treatment. *Fertil Steril* 2001;76: 461–8.

Thorneycroft, I. Evolution of progestins. Focus on the novel progestin drospirenone. *J Reprod Med* 2002;47(suppl 11):975–80.

Wysowsky DK, Pitts M, Beitz J. An analysis of reports of depression and suicide in patients treated with isotretinoin. *J Am Acad Dermatol* 2001;45:515–19.

van Vloten W, van Haselen CW, van Zuuren EJ et al. The effect of 2 combined oral contraceptives containing either drospirenone or cyproterone acetate on acne and seborrhea. *Cutis* 2002;69 (suppl 4):2–15.

Physical treatments for acne and scarring

Treatment of comedones and macrocomedones

Acne surgery involves expressing the contents of closed comedones in an effort to speed the resolution of acne. There are various types of comedone extractors, but each is a small instrument designed to apply pressure to the surface of the comedone to enucleate the cornified plug. There is a risk of increasing the inflammation associated with acne if the contents of the comedone are extruded into the dermis, rather than onto the surface of the skin. With the advent of effective topical retinoids, this procedure is used much less often.

Macrocomedones are large comedones that are often resistant to treatment with topical retinoids and oral isotretinoin. Use of light electrocautery 60–90 minutes after the application of the topical anesthetic EMLA on these lesions has been reported to accelerate their resolution.

Light. Sun exposure is reported to have a beneficial effect in up to 70% patients with acne. However, the effects are short-lived, and clearly the potential risk of skin malignancies negates the possible short-term improvement that UV light might induce in acne.

Recently, studies have examined the effect of visible light on acne, a treatment that has the advantage of avoiding the potential risks of UV radiation. *P. acnes* is known to produce endogenous porphyrins, which absorb visible light at 415 nm and could therefore produce a photodynamic reaction following irradiation with blue light. Red light is able to penetrate the tissue more deeply than blue light and has anti-inflammatory activity. A recent controlled study demonstrated significant improvement in inflammatory acne treated with combined blue–red light compared with white light and standard topical therapy. This study also demonstrated that combined blue–red light was better than red light alone. The light sources are portable and commercially available (Dermalux) and take 15 minutes per day to treat one site. This may represent a convenient therapy for some patients with mild-to-moderate acne.

Low-fluence pulsed-dye laser light has been used to treat a limited number of mild-to-moderate acne cases with good results, but further studies are needed to confirm these data.

Treatment of inflammatory nodules/cysts

The intralesional injection of corticosteroids such as triamcinolone can dramatically decrease the size of inflammatory cysts and nodules. Triamcinolone can be used in concentrations ranging from 2.5 to 10 mg/mL. Often a volume of 0.05 to 0.25 mL per lesion is used. Repeat injection after 3–4 weeks may be needed. This mode of therapy is a useful adjuvant to treatment with oral antibiotics or isotretinoin. It is particularly helpful in patients who develop these lesions only rarely and who are not candidates for treatment with isotretinoin.

Cryotherapy (two 5-second freeze–thaw cycles) may also be helpful in resistant cases.

Treatment of scars

The best solution to the problem of acne scarring is to institute appropriate therapy early in the course of acne to avoid this complication. Patients with a family history of scarring acne may be at increased risk of developing acne scars. Hypertrophic and keloidal scars occur most often on the chest and back of young patients with severe cystic acne. Referral to a dermatologist should be considered for a consultation regarding the possible use of intralesional injection with triamcinolone, treatment with silastic gel sheeting or laser therapy. Acne scars that are erythematous may respond to treatment with a pulsed-dye laser, which reduces the erythema of the scar. Successful treatment of atrophic acne scars with an erbium:YAG laser has recently been reported.

Ice-pick scars can be treated by selective excision with or without grafting, depending upon their size. Punch grafting is a useful technique wherein the scar is removed with a punch excision. The defect is then filled with a punch graft of normal skin from a donor area such as beneath the mastoid or posterior auricular area.

Dermabrasion or CO_2 laserbrasion can be used to improve facial acne scars that are shallow, papular or nodular. This procedure should only be performed after the patient's acne is no longer active. A waiting period of 6–12 months following treatment with isotretinoin is recommended before proceeding with dermabrasion; otherwise, patients can develop significant postinflammatory pigmentation.

Key points – physical treatment for acne and scarring

- Macrocomedones frequently require surgical treatment with cautery, as pharmacological therapeutic options are unhelpful.
- Acne nodules/cysts respond well to intralesional triamcinolone injection or cryotherapy.
- Acne scarring is common, and the best approach is prevention by early effective therapy.
- Laser therapy may be helpful for acne scarring.

Key references

Jacobs CI, Dover JS, Kaminer MS. Acne scarring: a classification system and review of treatment options. *J Am Acad Dermatol* 2001;45: 109–17.

Layton AM. Acne scarring – reviewing the need for early treatment of acne. *J Dermatol Treat* 2000; 11:3–6.

Papageorgiou P, Katsambas A, Chu A. Phototherapy with blue (415 nm) and red (660 nm) light in the treatment of acne vulgaris. *Br J Dermatol* 2000;142:973–8.

Seaton ED, Charakida A, Mouser PE et al. Pulsed-dye laser treatment for inflammatory acne vulgaris: randomised controlled trial. *Lancet* 2003;362:1347–52.

Thomson KF, Goulden V, Sheehan-Dare R, Cunliffe WJ. Light cautery of macrocomedones under general anaesthesia. *Br J Dermatol* 1999; 141:595–6.

Assessment

First, the overall severity of the patient's acne must be assessed. This should take account of clinical presentation (which may be graded with reference to a system such as that shown on pages 76–9), psychosocial effects, presence and potential for scarring, and by failure to respond to previous therapy. The type of topical treatment may be dictated by the predominant type of lesion, and for this reason good lighting is required in order to detect non-inflamed lesions, which can easily be missed otherwise. A one-page questionnaire, APSEA (Figure 8.1), is used by some doctors to assess the social and psychological effects of acne; others may use CADI or DQLI (see page 17).

Therapeutic approach

Patient discussion. A thorough discussion with the patient is necessary to dispel the myths about the disease. For example, food does not cause acne, acne is not infectious, and excessive washing does not influence the management of the disease. It needs to be stressed that acne is a chronic disease and that no response will be seen before a minimum of 4 weeks of therapy. This is especially important for teenage patients, who often become discouraged if results are not seen quickly despite the fact that they have been following their prescribed regimen. The patient must be told that if they have mild disease then topical treatment will be required, probably for 4 years, but up to 10–20 years if the disease is moderate or severe. In moderate and severe disease, oral therapies will be required for variable lengths of time. For example, oral antibiotics may be given for 6-monthly courses or longer, and if necessary the courses may be repeated for many years; an oral contraceptive may be prescribed for 2–5 years or longer, according to the women's contraceptive needs.

Pamphlets are available from the American Academy of Dermatology, the British Association of Dermatology, acne support groups and from some pharmaceutical companies that summarize the cause of the disease

Date: _____   Overall clinical grade of acne ☐ Mild ☐ Moderate ☐ Severe

Patient's Name: _____   APSEA score (value) _____

APSEA score (significance) ☐ Insig ☐ Low ☐ Mod ☐ High ☐ V.High

Question 1 to 6 please tick (✓) the box corresponding to the most appropriate answer

IN THE PAST WEEK

AT THE MOMENT

1. Worrying thoughts go through my mind
   ☐ a great deal
   ☐ a lot of the time
   ☐ from time to time
   ☐ only occasionally

4. I like what I look like in photographs
   ☐ not at all
   ☐ sometimes
   ☐ very often
   ☐ nearly all the time

2. I can sit at ease and feel relaxed
   ☐ definitely
   ☐ usually
   ☐ not often

5. I wish I looked better
   ☐ not at all
   ☐ sometimes
   ☐ very often

3. I feel restless, as if I have to be on the move
   ☐ very much indeed
   ☐ quite a lot
   ☐ not very much
   ☐ not at all

6. On the whole I am satisfied with myself
   ☐ strongly disagree
   ☐ disagree
   ☐ agree
   ☐ strongly agree

Question 7–9 – read the following carefully and put a mark at the point on the line that most accurately represents how you feel, e.g. _____/_____

7. I still enjoy the things I used to
   Never _____ All the time

8. I am more irritable than usual
   Never _____ All the time

9. I feel that I am useful and needed
   Never _____ All the time

Question 10–15 – How does the present state of your skin condition limit the following activities or make them more difficult or awkward or less enjoyable – once again please put a mark at the point on the line, e.g. _____/_____

10. Going shopping
    Not at all _____ All the time

11. Going out socially to meet friends from outside the home
    Not at all _____ All the time

12. Going away for weekends, holidays and outings
    Not at all _____ All the time

13. Eating out
    Not at all _____ All the time

14. Using public changing rooms/swimming pools
    Not at all _____ All the time

15. Do you think your appearance will interfere with your chances of future employment?
    Strongly disagree _____ Strongly agree

Figure 8.1 The APSEA questionnaire for the assessment of social and psychological effects

and the principles of its treatment. Such handouts are helpful, but are not a substitute for an adequate discussion with the patient.

Rationale for selection of appropriate antiacne agents. Figure 8.2 gives an algorithm for the selection of treatment options once the patient's overall acne severity has been assessed to be mild, moderate or severe. In all cases, the choice of a specific agent or agents should seek to achieve maximum efficacy and tolerability with minimum risk of adverse effects. For non-inflammatory acne, or for mild-to-moderate inflammatory acne, topical therapy may be sufficient, and this minimizes potential adverse effects associated with the use of systemic agents. Moderate-to-severe inflammatory disease not responding to topical combination therapy warrants the addition of oral agents to the regimen. In designing a topical therapeutic regimen, attention to the specific formulations available is warranted. Existing preparations of some topical agents can cause significant local irritation, which decreases tolerability and may, therefore, decrease compliance, particularly in teenage males who are not accustomed to applying creams or lotions to their faces.

Rational use of combination therapy in the management of acne requires consideration of the pathogenic factors involved and an understanding of how the various antiacne agents target one or more of these factors. Regimens should be designed to take advantage of the synergistic effects of agents with different mechanisms of action that can target a combination of the pathogenic factors associated with acne.

Poor response to therapy

The major reasons for poor response to conventional antibiotic therapy are outlined in Table 8.1. The commonest of these is an inadequate amount of therapy because of poor compliance, inadequate instructions or the failure to emphasize to the patient the need for long-term and continued therapy provided there are no side effects and progress is adequate. The side effects (see pages 41 and 52) will obviously interfere with the rate of progress, but many alternative therapies are usually possible. Resistance of *P. acnes* is becoming an

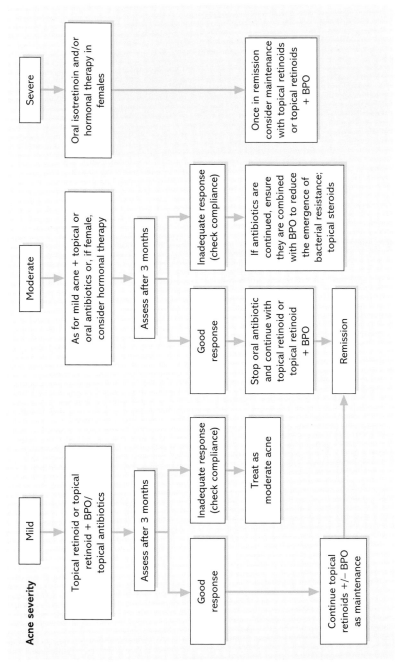

Figure 8.2 Algorithm for acne therapy. BPO, benzoyl peroxide.

TABLE 8.1

Reasons for poor therapeutic response to antibiotics

- Incorrect use of the treatment by the patient, because of inadequate instructions or poor compliance
- Inadequate potency (e.g. dose too low)
- Folliculitis due to staphylococci, Gram-negative enterobacteria or *Malassezia*
- Antibiotic-resistant *P. acnes*

increasing reason for poor response. In 1975 there was no resistant *P. acnes*. Now, in a specialized teaching clinic (Leeds, UK), resistance is detected in 67% of patients referred; the figure in primary care is on the order of 25%. However, the relationship between the presence of high levels of resistance and clinical failure is not clear cut. The reason for this is that if the drug concentration in the follicle is higher than the minimum inhibitory concentration of *P. acnes* then the patient will respond. Furthermore, some antibiotics such as minocycline have anti-inflammatory action independent of their effect on *P. acnes*. However, it is likely that in about 25% of patients who have microbiological evidence of resistant *P. acnes*, this finding is clinically relevant.

Unfortunately it is not easy to grow *P. acnes*, and thus some overall guidelines are necessary to allow the physician to suspect, prevent and treat *P. acnes* resistance (Table 8.2). *P. acnes* resistance should be suspected in patients who are not responding, patients who were responding but relapse, and those who have had multiple courses of different topical and oral antibiotics. The treatment of suspected *P. acnes* resistance includes the use of those antibiotics for which there is less evidence of resistance as yet, such as oral trimethoprim and minocycline, and the use of a higher rather than a lower dose of a topical antibiotic, such as 4% concentration rather than 2%. Likewise, higher oral doses of therapy may be indicated, such as 200 mg of minocycline or 600 mg of trimethoprim. Some preparations, such as non-antibiotic

TABLE 8.2

Antibiotic resistance of _Propionibacterium acnes_

Reasons to suspect resistance

- Primary therapeutic failure: failure to respond to 4-month course of antibiotic
- Secondary therapeutic failure: relapse after therapy that was initially successful

Preventing resistance

- Only use antibiotics when necessary and for defined periods
- Use a non-antibiotic antimicrobial in conjunction with topical antibiotics and between antibiotic courses
- Use adequate doses of oral antibiotics
- If relapse occurs after stopping antibiotic, restart the same antibiotic type
- Encourage compliance
- Avoid cross-contamination between doctor and patient

Management of suspected resistance

- Skin swab and culture to detect resistant strains
- Consider topical non-antibiotic antimicrobials, topical or systemic retinoids, hormone treatments
- Consider increasing dose of oral antibiotic
- Avoid changing antibiotic

antimicrobials, i.e. benzoyl peroxide and topical retinoids, will never be associated with _P. acnes_ resistance, nor will oral contraceptives or oral isotretinoin.

Referral or consultation guidelines
Referral or consultation may be considered for:
- patients who may require treatment with isotretinoin for acne fulminans, severe inflammatory, cystic or scarring acne, recalcitrant comedonal acne, or Gram-negative folliculitis

- female patients whose acne may be associated with an endocrine disorder
- patients with acne scarring
- pregnant patients with acne.

Prevention

Early treatment of acne is likely, although not proven, to prevent or further modify development of the disease, and thus the early use of appropriate topical therapy in mild acne may well prevent development of moderate acne. Early treatment of siblings of already established patients is an area where this approach may prove most beneficial.

Key points – designing an acne treatment plan

- A clinical history must be carefully taken, including family history, previous treatments and response to therapy.
- The patient must be carefully examined, noting acne lesion type, extent and severity as well as acne scarring.
- Patients need to have realistic expectations and need to be able to comply with prescribed therapy.
- Prescribers should be aware of the emergence of antibiotic-resistant *Propionibacterium acnes*.
- Early effective therapy reduces the significant clinical and psychological morbidity associated with acne.

Key reference

Katsambas AD. Why and when the treatment of acne fails. *Dermatology* 1998;196:158–61.

In all situations, the primary goal of acne treatment is maximization of efficacy while minimizing the risk of adverse effects and scarring. In the management of acne, a variety of established therapies with different mechanisms of action are available to accomplish this goal. However, successful treatment with these agents is sometimes limited by tolerability or resistance problems. For example, topical retinoids are often associated with local irritation which can present a compliance problem for a number of patients. Benzoyl peroxide is also a local irritant and can bleach clothing. Topical and systemic antimicrobial agents may sometimes lose efficacy because of the development of resistant strains of *P. acnes*. In addition, oral antimicrobial agents are associated with systemic adverse effects, primarily gastrointestinal in nature, that can contribute to decreased efficacy because of reduced compliance. Finally, isotretinoin is associated with a number of systemic adverse effects, the most significant of which is teratogenicity. Consequently, there is ample opportunity for new antiacne agents to contribute to our ability to safely and effectively manage this chronic disease.

Research can contribute to our understanding of the pathophysiology of acne. Such an understanding will facilitate the development of more effective acne therapies. For example, great strides are being made in retinoid research. As we learn more about the interaction of retinoids with the various retinoid receptors and the sequence of subsequent cellular responses, we may increase our understanding of the mechanisms involved in the development of follicular hyperkeratinization.

Apart from hormonal therapy and systemic isotretinoin, little can be done to reduce sebum production. There is a clear need in acne therapy for better agents to inhibit sebum production. Sebum production is thought to be modulated in part by the androgen dihydrotestosterone (stanolone). This hormone is produced from testosterone by the action of the 5α-reductase enzyme. Research into the factors regulating sebum production will improve our understanding of this process and may lead to the identification of new therapeutic target sites. For example, two isozymes of 5α-reductase have been identified. The type 1 isozyme predominates in human sebaceous glands. If specific inhibitors of this isozyme can be developed that are safe and effective in reducing sebum production, these compounds may then constitute a novel class of future antiacne agents.

New anti-inflammatory agents, such as 5-lipoxygenase inhibitors, represent an interesting field of research. Preliminary clinical data are now available.

Clinically, dermatologists have been aware of the development of antibiotic resistance in patients whose initial favorable response to antibiotics waned over time. Traditionally, antibiotics were periodically switched in an effort to regain control over the patient's acne. Additional epidemiological studies are needed to track patterns of *P. acnes* resistance to antibiotics. Data gained from such studies will aid in the development of guidelines for designing therapeutic regimens that can minimize the development of resistance.

Key references

Cunliffe WJ. Looking back to the future – Acne. *Dermatology* 2002; 204:167–72.

Daniel F, Dreno B, Taieb A. Synthèse et proposition de travaux ulterieurs. *Ann Dermatol Vénéréol* 2001;128: 2S35–6.

Thiboutot D. New treatments and therapeutic strategies for acne. *Arch Fam Med* 2000;9:179–87.

Zouboulis C, Nestoris S, Adler Y et al. A new concept for acne therapy: a pilot study with zileuton, an oral 5-lipoxygenase inhibitor. *Arch Dermatol* 2003;139:668–70.

Zouboulis C, Piquero-Martin J. Update and future of systemic acne treatment. *Dermatology* 2003;206: 37–53.

The Leeds Acne Grading System

These examples from the Leeds Acne Grading System show facial acne varying in severity from least (grade 1) to greatest (grade 12), plus an example of nodulocystic acne. The grading is based on the number of inflamed lesions and their inflammatory intensity.

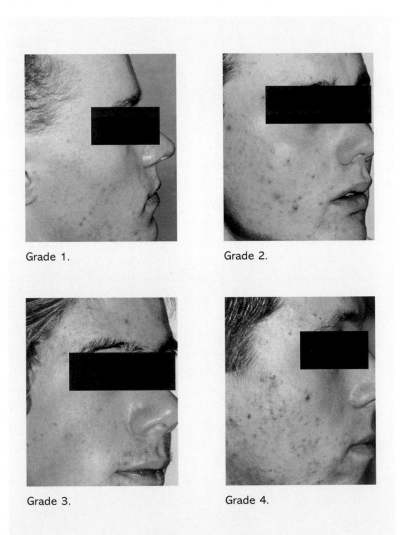

Grade 1.

Grade 2.

Grade 3.

Grade 4.

The Leeds Acne Grading System (continued)

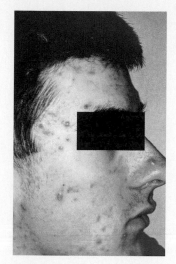

Grade 5.

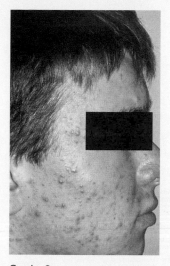

Grade 6.

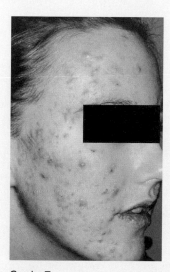

Grade 7.

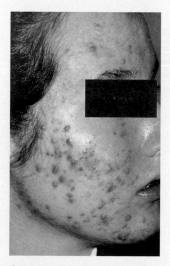

Grade 8.

The Leeds Acne Grading System (continued)

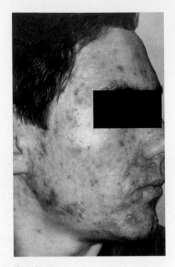

Grade 9.

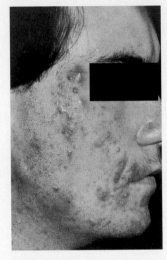

Grade 10.

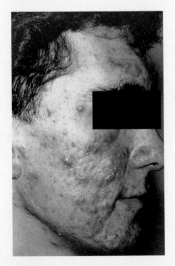

Grade 11.

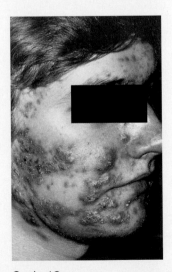

Grade 12.

The Leeds Acne Grading System (continued)

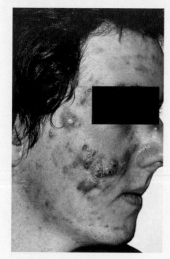

Grade nodulocystic acne

Useful addresses

Acne Support Group
PO Box 9, Newquay
Cornwall TR9 6WG, UK
Tel: 0870 870 2263
www.m2w3.com/acne/
www.stopspots.org (for teenagers)

British Red Cross Skin Camouflage Service
9 Grosvenor Crescent
London SW1X 7EJ, UK

Changing Faces
1 & 2 Junction Mews, Paddington
London W2 1PN, UK
phone: 020 7706 4232
fax: 020 7706 4234
info@changingfaces.co.uk
www.changingfaces.co.uk

National Library of Medicine, USA
www.nlm.nih.gov/medlineplus/acne.html

AcneNet
(sponsored by Roche Pharmaceuticals in collaboration with the
American Academy of Dermatology)
www.derm-infonet.com/acnenet

Index

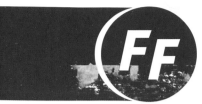

FAST FACTS

Acne

*Indispensable
Guides to
Clinical
Practice*

Alison M Layton MB ChB MRCP
Consultant Dermatologist
Harrogate District Hospital
Harrogate, UK

Diane Thiboutot MD
Associate Professor of Dermatology
Pennsylvania State University College of Medicine
Hershey, Pennsylvania, USA

Vincenzo Bettoli MD
Assistant Professor
Department of Dermatology
University of Ferrara, Italy

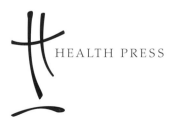

HEALTH PRESS

Oxford

Fast Facts – Acne
First published January 2004
Text © 2004 Alison M Layton, Diane Thiboutot, Vincenzo Bettoli

© 2004 in this edition Health Press Limited
Health Press Limited, Elizabeth House, Queen Street, Abingdon,
Oxford OX14 3JR, UK
Tel: +44 (0)1235 523233
Fax: +44 (0)1235 523238

Fast Facts is a trademark of Health Press Limited.

Alison Layton is grateful to Professor William Cunliffe for advice and the
provision of some illustrations.

ISBN 1-899541-73-X

Layton, AM (Alison)
Fast Facts – Acne/
Alison M Layton, Diane Thiboutot, Vincenzo Bettoli

Medical illustrations by Dee McLean, London, UK.
Typesetting and page layout by Zed, Oxford, UK.
Printed by Fine Print (Services) Ltd, Oxford, UK.

Printed with vegetable inks on fully biodegradable and
recyclable paper manufactured from sustainable forests.

Low emissions
during production

Low
chlorine

Sustainable
forests